Introduction

I'm no doctor, nor do I have any kind of degree related to the subject matter of this book. However, I was an adjunct professor for ten years at Miami-Dade Community College and trained certified computer repair technicians.

While the problems and solutions of malfunctioning computers have nothing in common with those of "malfunctioning" people, the troubleshooting method is exactly the same: identify the problem, identify the cause, identify the solution, and apply the solution.

Although I have no credentials in the health profession, I am a consumer and I found myself looking down the massive vitamins and supplements aisle of a typical drug store and realized that there was absolutely no way a person could walk up, pick a vitamin off the shelf, and get it right.

Furthermore, I realized that there was no way anyone could pick ANY product off of those shelves and get it right – that is, try to take something that would shore up what they perceive to be their weakness. And how could a person, like myself, even know what their weaknesses were in the first place?

This series of books intends to address this problem. I have done all of the research and I can tell you exactly which products have the best ingredients – which ones work – and which ones are appropriate. And I can warn you which ones have such useless ingredients in them that they are worth avoiding.

While I originally set out to deal specifically with the dietary supplement market and its products, I realized that nutrition is a much wider subject and that these products are not the issue at all: achieving OPTIMUM THRIVE-LEVEL health and maintaining that, is, or should be, the primary focus of everyone. Therefore the big question is: how is this done?

One in three Americans will die of cancer, and hundreds of thousands die each year from heart disease. These top 2 causes of death in the U.S. kill over 1.2 MILLION people accounting for 45% of ALL deaths each year in the U.S. and those numbers are on the rise.[167] Even with all of our amazing advances in medical science, things are getting worse, not better. And there is a reason for this: POOR DIET and LACK of EXERCISE.

Three things are killing people:

1. CANCER CAUSING ADDITIVES in PROCESSED foods: Many people eat these POISONS on a DAILY BASIS. And they are exposed to other POISONS like DIESEL ENGINE FUMES, HARSH CLEANER FUMES, etc.)

2. POOR DIET: even if you eat good foods, an unmanaged diet consisting of nothing but natural whole foods will most likely fail to deliver everything the body needs because some nutrients are rare in the plant kingdom and only a few foods actually provide them in significant quantities. Without knowing precisely what the body needs and what foods can fulfill those needs, a person will suffer chronic deficiencies in critical nutrients which can have severe consequences to their health.

3. LACK OF EXERCISE: You cannot expect to be healthy if you do not engage in EXERCISE. Exercise is necessary for cardiovascular health and sweating is one of the methods the body uses for detoxification, therefore it is vital for OPTIMUM THRIVE-LEVEL health.

This series is designed to explain the needs of the human body and how to cover those needs in order to achieve OPTIMUM THRIVE-LEVEL health and avoid the BIG SEVEN modern deadly epidemic plagues that are killing over a MILLION people each year: 1) High Blood Pressure, 2) High Cholesterol, 3) Type II Diabetes, 4) Alzheimer's Disease, 5) Cardiovascular Disease, 6) Stroke and 7) Cancer. Why isn't "heart attack" in the Big Seven? Heart failure is most certainly in there: it is final event of High Blood Pressure, High Cholesterol and Cardiovascular Disease. It is important to know that the primary cause of ALL of these modern plagues is POOR DIET and that MOST of those deaths are PREVENTABLE.

Most people scoff at Natural Whole Foods and Medicinal Herbs. However, the vast majority of ALL drugs from Over-The-Counter medications like Aspirin – the top selling drug of all time, to Morphine – a Class 1 Controlled substance, were originally discovered in plants; Aspirin was discovered in Willow Bark Tea used by Native Americans and Morphine was isolated from the latex of fresh Poppy plant seed pods. And although science has identified hundreds of compounds in every plant that has been analyzed, they still contain possibly hundreds more that have yet to be identified. That's tens of thousands of known substances MOST of which have never been studied for their potential health benefits and possibly MILLIONS that have yet to be discovered.

Although the research has only just begun in earnest, science has already verified the enormous health promoting power of hundreds of edible plants and hundreds more medicinal plants and there is no reason to doubt that they can and will provide not only the well known and thoroughly tested vitamins and minerals, but also their own unique spectrum of phytonutrients that can help prevent just about every possible affliction and provide effective treatment for most of them as well; including and especially the BIG SEVEN modern deadly epidemic plagues.

.

In the case of the Natural Whole Food and Holistic Herbs Diet, one might assume that there is no physiological problem to identify and fix, but that is not necessarily true. If the goal is to live a longer, healthier and happier life and avoid the BIG SEVEN modern deadly epidemics, then it is important to realize that the body is a machine and it has maintenance requirements. We do fight off most microbes and we heal from most injuries on our own. A doctor might place your leg in a cast simply to immobilize it, but our own bones or rather the cells in them, are well aware of the problem and begin to grow and multiply and rebuild the region at the site of the break as quickly as they can. So the doctor doesn't heal the broken bone, our own bodies do that work. And as long as the cells are getting ALL of the raw materials necessary to get this work done, then it will always get done. However, even when there is no disease or injury, cells continuously die and have to be replaced. We get a whole new skin – the single largest organ of the human body, by the way – every 35 days on average. That requires a lot of raw building materials ranging from amino acids that are the bricks used to build the cell walls made up of proteins, along with plenty of fuel in the form of calories to get that work done, and virtually ALL of the "Big 43" essential nutrients (the vitamins, minerals, and a few others) are required for this work to get done as well.

But the Big 43 are only the beginning of the ESSENTIAL nutrient requirements. Discoveries are being made every year that indicate that potentially hundreds of other compounds found primarily in the plants are also required for OPTIMUM THRIVE-LEVEL health. And the skin is not the only organ that undergoes this constant rollover of cells dying and being replaced; virtually all organs in the human body have cells that are continuously dying and being replaced to some lesser or greater extent.

So if OPTIMUM THRIVE-LEVEL health is the goal, and the human body has the largest and most complex set of nutritional requirements of any life form on Earth, then there IS a problem: most people are only vaguely aware that they need the vitamins which are easy to remember for the most part, and some minerals, but few are aware that Selenium, Chromium, Manganese and Molybdenum, to cite just a few, are ESSENTIAL nutrients too. And an unmanaged diet (eating whatever whenever) even if it consists almost entirely of natural whole foods, cannot possibly provide you with ALL of the "Big 43" in the ideal amounts that the body needs on a regular basis. And if any ONE of those essential nutrients falls short over a long period of time, then it becomes an issue and in some cases will lead to disease and even death if the deficiency is allowed to continue. So if the problem begins with poor diet, then correcting the diet is a good place to start.

THE NATURAL WHOLE FOODS DIET

I can actually divide this up into the MAIN HEALTHY FOOD GROUPS. These differ dramatically from the food groups that we grew up with for one reason: those food groups were established back during the Great Depression and had everything to do with supporting the farmers so they could pay the mortgages on their properties and keep the banks from collapsing, and they had to do with popular beliefs about the foods and had almost nothing to do with SCIENCE.

THE GOOD FOODS LIST – PRIMARY FOODS

The definition of the "Primary Food" group is: those foods that can be eaten fresh and raw. Edible raw foods raised up early man for millions of years from whatever he was, to what he is now. Only within the last 100,000 years, more or less, did man tame fire and accidentally discover cooking. Therefore any food that can be eaten raw, is in the Primary Food Group, even if you do choose to cook it. All meats are edible raw, but doing that is certainly NOT RECOMMENDED. Cooking animal meats makes sure that any unwelcome microbes, microscopic eggs, or larvae will be killed. I had the honor of being taught my freshman Biology class by Dr. Goldberg who was a marine biologist whose main interest was parasitic worms. He presented weeks of hour long slide shows of fish he had caught and splayed open revealing them to be packed literally to the gills with worms of every color of the rainbow and more different sizes and shapes than us Italians have for pasta: one fish contained nothing but corkscrew shaped gray ones, another was nothing but egg noodle shaped orange ones under the skin, the next was completely packed full of spaghetti-shaped red ones… meat is a Primary Food, but be sure to COOK IT THOROUGHLY. (I still nightmare about those images and merely suggesting Sushi to me will result in a long winded tirade.)

1) EDIBLE RAW VEGETABLES – Anything that can be eaten raw including all of the green leafy vegetables from lettuce and cabbage and their kin, to celery, to carrots, to onions, to broccoli are all exceptionally healthy foods loaded with essential nutrients as well as their own phytonutrients currently under investigation and being proven in studies to have enormous health benefits. .

2) FRUITS – The vast majority are loaded with Vitamin C along with many other essential nutrients including antioxidants that have been shown to provide significant health benefits.

3) NUTS – These are loaded with Vitamin E and many different minerals depending on the type of nut. Although they are high in fat, it is the good kind, polyunsaturated fat, but they still pack a lot of calories and are not the best friend to anyone trying to control or lose weight.

4) SEEDS – Sunflower seeds are the KING of the SEED foods. They are a SUPERFOOD and highly recommended. Pumpkin seeds and many others are also loaded with essential nutrients and are highly recommended as well. However, like the nuts, they are very high in polyunsaturated fats and therefore calories.

5) YOGURT – This is a very healthy alternative to ice cream. You can buy it plain and add your own fruits, nuts and seeds to it or buy it with the fruits already added, just check the ingredients label and make sure there are no artificial chemical additives. Yogurt is high in Calcium and excellent for your health.[46]

6) FISH – Mackerel, Salmon, Sardines, Cod, and Tuna are all loaded with essential nutrients, but ALL fish and other sea foods are very healthy foods and excellent sources of Complete Protein and they are the ONLY sources of the Omega-3 fatty acids DHA (Docosahexaenoic acid) and EPA (Eicosapentaenoic acid) that our bodies need.

7) FRUIT AND VEGETABLE JUICES – Replace soda pop and other junk beverages with these healthy alternatives. ALL vegetable juices MUST be the "Low Sodium" versions. These use potassium salts to make them salty rather than sodium salts. Our bodies NEED HUGE quantities of Potassium to ensure proper function of the nerve endings for muscle activation, proper electrolyte balance, and proper fluid osmotic pressure throughout the body. Chronic low potassium is likely the number one cause of High Blood Pressure which can lead to heart failure which is the number one cause of death in the United States today. Low Sodium vegetable juice contains about 23% of the U. S. Food and Drug Administration's Recommended Daily Allowance (RDA) of Potassium in an 8 ounce cup and drinking three such servings per day will lower blood pressure, SAVE YOUR HEART, and your life.

8) SPICES – While we don't actually sit down to a bowl of cloves for lunch, most spices pack a powerful punch, not just in flavor but also in antioxidant power and phytonutrients. They get their strong aromas and flavors from these compounds, many of which are currently under investigation for their well known powerful health benefits including preventing high blood pressure, high cholesterol, cardiovascular disease and heart attack, and even actively fighting cancer. Adding a bunch of these to everything you cook can and will lead to better health (and tastier food too!)

THE BAD FOODS LIST

While correcting your diet you must avoid the following:

1) NO PACKAGED AND/OR PROCESSED FOODS – This includes100% Whole Grain bread. Get this from the local bakery with NO ADDED CHEMICALS, NO HIGH FRUCTOSE CORN SYRUP, and ABSOLUTELY NEVER any HYDROGENATED (or "hydrolyzed") VEGETABLE OIL of any kind. All three of these along with processed white cane sugar are PROVEN irritants of the liver that have been shown to cause high blood pressure, high cholesterol, diabetes and CANCER.

2) NO SOY or its BY-PRODUCTS: These are CHEAP GARBAGE FILLERS in virtually all processed and packaged foods that they won't even feed to cows, goats or pigs. If it's not good enough for them, why are they giving it to us? Many studies are starting to show that chronic overindulgence of soy beans and their by-products can be TOXIC to humans and this CRUD is definitely TOXIC to grazing animals: enough said. If you are drinking soy milk I urge you to consider Almond milk or some other alternative.

3) NO "FORTIFIED" or "ENRICHED" foods. The added vitamins and minerals are always synthetic and inferior quality; some might actually be TOXIC.

4) NO MAYONNAISE or its KIN: This includes creamy salad dressings and creamy dips which are all made with raw egg which is BAD FOR YOU. Raw egg binds with Vitamin B7 – Biotin in particular, but it could also block the absorption of the other B vitamins to some extent: you don't need this stuff in your digestive tract BLOCKING the absorption of the B Vitamins that you NEED and are PAYING FOR and PAYING ATTENTION TO specifically in order to get them. Drop these foods forever.

5) NO PROCESSED MEATS: No: hotdogs, sausages, bacon, "Luncheon meat" (i.e. "Spam") "Potted meat" (i.e. "Deviled Ham") etc. Jerky and kippered meats add too much plain SALT (no Iodine) and NITRITES as preservatives which are DREADFUL POISONS to the liver.

6) NO SODA POP – Most of these nuisances contain NOTHING THAT WAS EVER ALIVE. The mild carbonic acid which gives them their fizz, is BAD FOR YOUR DIGESTIVE TRACT and most are laced with artificial colors and flavors. (They don't really need preservatives because even the bacteria want no part of them!) Eliminate this GARBAGE from your diet. Drink vegetable and fruit juices instead as well as plenty of water which is the number one liquid ESSENTIAL NUTRIENT you can drink for better health and it also helps lower blood pressure.

7) NO CANDY – This crud is ALL terrible. Eat fruits instead. Many are just as sweet as candy but contain FRUCTOSE which is a very healthy form of sugar that your body does need to function. Your brain runs on glucose; no sugar = pass out. Ask anyone suffering from hypoglycemia or diabetes and they can tell you all about it. Fructose must be converted into glucose which SLOWS DOWN its absorption and arrival in the blood stream. This gives many fruits a lower "Glycemic Index" than expected which is a measurement of how strongly and quickly foods impact blood sugar levels.

8) FAST FOOD/JUNK FOOD: Most of these foods are low in nutritional value and high in saturated fat, cholesterol and calories and cause weight gain, high cholesterol, high blood pressure and therefore increase the risk of serious cardiovascular disease and have also been linked to increased risk of diabetes and cancer.

9) BAKED GOODS – Most are based on bleached white wheat flour which is NOTHING BUT GLUTEN with almost no nutritional value, and they are also loaded with processed white cane sugar which has been shown to cause Type II Diabetes, increase blood pressure, irritate the liver and increase the risk of cancer. Many such products are now made with enriched flour which is a joke; 100% whole wheat flour is loaded with nutrients because the wheat germ has been kept in the creation of the flour. By removing it, they have to go back and add vitamins and minerals which are always synthetic and of inferior quality making the entire process a ridiculous exercise and effectively turning what could have been a good food into a bad one loaded with MORE manmade chemicals.

THE SECONDARY FOODS THAT SHOULD BE DRAMATICALLY REDUCED IN A HEALTHY DIET

1) GRAINS – Most people think I am a lunatic when I call these BAD FOODS, and they are certainly not totally evil, but anything that has to be cooked in order to become edible is definitely on the SECONDARY FOOD list which means you should not eat them regularly as a group. Foods made from processed grains like white flour are a definite PROBLEM and are BAD FOR YOU. I apologize to all of the bakers out there, but bleached processed white flour donuts, pastries and cookies sweetened with processed white cane sugar are nothing but trash calories and DEADLY and mess with your liver and you must avoid them. Bleached wheat flour products, corn and rice (especially milled white rice) are the primary culprits and should be significantly reduced in your weekly dietary regimen. Most of these foods have astronomical Glycemic Index scores and irritate the liver and the blood sugar regulatory system. There are a few exceptions to each rule: see the list of exceptions to the rules below.

2) STARCHY ROOTS – Anything that must be cooked in order to make it edible including potatoes, yucca, malanga, boniato, etc. I know this is bad news for a lot of people and trust me I miss them sorely too, but the truth is that these foods are high in calories of the worst kind: starches that when cooked result in foods with Glycemic Index scores HIGHER than HONEY. And while a few may bring some essential nutrients, it is not enough to justify the irritation they cause the liver and blood sugar regulatory system. Eat them very sparingly.

3) BEANS – Kidney, Navy, Pinto, etc are all SECONDARY FOODS: eat them sparingly. Most beans are high in "crude fiber" so they must be soaked then boiled for long periods of time to make them edible. It is this form of fiber that causes "digestive difficulties." The body is trying to tell you not to eat them, so don't.

SOME FOODS (SHOULD BE REDUCED) THAT ARE NOT SO EVIL AS YOU THINK

1) EGGS – Maligned for decades since the discovery of the link between cholesterol and heart disease, eggs are NOT going to kill you unless you eat them raw or by the dozen. I have three eggs for breakfast about once a week. However, my cholesterol is under control. If yours is high you should stay away until you have it under control and PLEASE do not take those terrible drugs to do it. A proper diet can correct this modern epidemic which is not really even a disease, but a symptom – of POOR DIET.

2) DAIRY – I realize that this is a SECONDARY FOOD and many people are developing lactose intolerance. This is due mainly to OVERINDULGENCE and its presence in far too great a quantity in the average modern diet. Cheese and even REAL butter are far healthier than products based on HYDROGENATED VEGETABLE OIL – that junk is artificial animal fat and the liver doesn't know what to do with it: it irritates the liver and that is trouble. By the way, I know a lot of people that have switched to 2% skim milk or even 1% and 0% (which tastes like white colored water to me.) Do you know the percentage of fat content in whole milk? Most people guess 20% to 50% when I ask them this question and I have to laugh. Do you realize that Half and Half has this percentage of fat? "Whole milk" is an advertising term that arose when people started to complain because the milk had all of the cream removed when it was pasteurized and homogenized and to them (back then) it tasted like 0% skim milk tastes to me now. Modern "Whole milk" which has had most of the cream removed is about 3% to 5%. They aren't going to leave much in it because they can sell it in the form of cheese, butter and other products at a premium.

3) POULTRY – Chicken and turkey meat (skinned to remove a lot of the fats and cholesterol) are the second healthiest source of animal protein (Fish are by far #1) that you can eat and should be part of your regular weekly eating regimen… just DON'T FRY IT!

4) BEEF – Often blamed for causing high cholesterol as well, beef is also not nearly as evil as people now believe. Beef is high in many essential nutrients and the only source of some essential amino acids for most people unless they also eat poultry and fish. Beef liver, which is an organ, and not the beef meat, is one of nature's true SUPERFOODS and it is LOADED with vitamins and minerals and is excellent for you (even though it makes me gag.)

5) PORK – Well trimmed choice cuts of FRESH Pork are not as evil as you might believe. It actually brings a very good ratio of the nine essential amino acids as well as Vitamin B3, B6, Selenium and Zinc in excellent amounts.

SECONDARY FOODS THAT ARE
NOTABLE EXCEPTIONS TO THE RULES

1) OATMEAL – Even though this is a grain and would normally be considered a SECONDARY FOOD (to be eaten very sparingly) OATMEAL happens to be an excellent "preventative" food for the heart. Because it promotes heart health by lowering cholesterol, I advise oatmeal as the only cereal to eat for breakfast. Stick to "old-fashioned" oats rather than "instant" because the instant has been processed in some way in order to make it instant. True old-fashioned oatmeal is the food that is good for your heart. Aside from the Vitamin B1, Magnesium, Molybdenum, Manganese and

Selenium that it brings, it is also high in Dietary Fiber and contains Beta-Glucans, complex forms of sugar also found in very high quantities in edible mushrooms that have numerous studies showing that they are powerful immunostimulants and also help fight certain forms of cancer.[155]

2) BUCKWHEAT – Buckwheat is a Net Negative Calorie Food, surprising for a seed (it is not a true grain.) And it is an excellent breakfast alternative.

3) TEFF – Teff is not well known in the U.S. but I am sure its day is coming; it is the only true grain in the Net Negative Calorie Foods (right around 29 cal/oz) and it is the lowest calorie true grain that I can find. Any goods baked with Teff flour will have at least 25% LESS CALORIES than those made from other grain flours.

4) THE LEGUMES – CHICKPEAS, GREEN PEAS, LENTILS, BLACKEYE PEAS and PEANUTS are excellent sources of Dietary Fiber and many essential nutrients that are difficult to get from other foods like Molybdenum. Some are also surprisingly low in calories like Green Peas, while Lentils have over 10 TIMES the antioxidant power of raw carrots. Peanuts are loaded with nutrients but they are rather high in calories. Peanut Oil might not be the healthiest oil (Coconut is #1, and the rest are in order are: Olive, Sesame, Safflower, Sunflower, and Canola, all others are to be AVOIDED) nevertheless, foods cooked in peanut oil take on a great flavor and I add a little on occasion to tap into that wonderful taste and aroma.

5) THE HEALTHY BEANS - LIMA, BLACK, FAVA, SNAP, MUNG and GREEN BEANS – All of these beans are true SECONDARY FOODS, however each one brings Dietary Fiber, some essential nutrients and/or specific phytonutrients with health promoting properties and they are all Net Negative Calorie Foods (less than 30 cal/oz.) making them excellent choices for a healthy diet..

THE BASIC NATURAL WHOLE FOODS DIET FOR OPTIMUM HEALTH

The primary focus is obviously to eat as many natural whole foods as possible rather than packaged and processed foods loaded with trash calories and laced with chemicals most of which have already been shown in many studies to be CANCER-CAUSING POISONS..

The problem with the natural whole foods diet is that many items actually have a lot of calories, most heavy plant foods like Sesame Seed Butter (a.k.a. Tahini,) Avocado, and Chocolate (100% Pure Cacao) are loaded with polyunsaturated fats. These are the "good kind" and they are also loaded with fat-soluble phytonutrients of enormous health benefit like Vitamin E and the Omega-6 fatty acids. And some are loaded with alpha-Linoleic Acid which is the only Omega-3 fatty acid found in plants (in reasonable amounts.)

Since seeds and nuts are the primary culprits of bringing large

9

amounts of polyunsaturated fats and therefore calories, it would seem that in order to avoid gaining weight, these heavy plant foods should be reduced in serving sizes on a daily basis. .

And if that is true, then there are many essential nutrients found primarily in the seeds and nuts that would be missing or in reduced amounts in the other foods and that would mean that they would have to come from supplements instead of natural sources.

Also there are several members of the "Big 43" essential nutrients that are very difficult to get from an exclusively natural whole foods diet even if it is under no caloric limitations. Choline and Calcium are particularly problematic if a person has to avoid dairy products (lactose intolerance) or is trying to avoid weight gain and is refraining from foods high in saturated fat and cholesterol.

If the goal is to achieve OPTIMUM THRIVE-LEVEL health and to avoid eating excessive calories, then it is necessary to develop a managed diet. There are too many foods that are, to be blunt: "Nonfunctional." They bring plenty of calories but little in the way of nutritional value. And when those foods that do bring significant nutritional value are added, many of them also bring a significant amount of calories as well. Therefore the nonfunctional foods must be replaced by the Functional foods; those that may bring calories, but they are worth it because they also bring significant amounts of the essential nutrients that the body must have on a daily basis to function properly and maintain OPTIMUM THRIVE-LEVEL health.

The human body absorbs matter from the environment in order to function – to survive. We need in order of priority: Oxygen, Water, Calories, Protein (the Nine Essential Amino Acids), followed by the rest of the "Big 43" essential nutrients, and finally the micronutrients and the phytonutrients found in plants. If a person gets plenty of the first four but falls short of the rest of the Big 43 essential nutrients, they could survive for months perhaps even years, but their health will gradually decline and they will get sick and eventually die. Even getting all of the Big 43 in proper amounts is not perfect either because we still do not know how much of the remaining micronutrients and phytonutrients that the body also needs. But we do know that many trace minerals are found in the human body and that many of these are also found in plants. Since we are the descendants of Hunter-Gatherers that survived primarily on edible raw plant foods for millions of years, it stands to reason that we need some of these same nutrients in trace amounts as well.

The bottom line here is to pursue a varied diet, centered on foods low in calories, and to make certain that we get those Big 43 essential nutrients and that we are also getting a variety of plant foods that can provide the trace micronutrients and the enormous variety of phytochemicals which science is currently studying and discovering that they possess a wide range of health promoting powers as well.

10

THE NATURAL WHOLE FOODS DIET

1) THE "NET NEGATIVE CALORIE" FOODS – All of these foods have very low calories: less than 30 cal/oz. If every food you eat all day contained 25 cal/oz, then you would have to eat 80 oz total to get 2000 calories for the day – that's FIVE POUNDS of food which very few people could eat. Cucumbers contain about 3.3 cal/oz. and it would take 36 pounds of them to reach 2000 calories and no one can eat that much in a day. Some NNC Foods: **Watercress** (Raw, Chopped 3.7cal/cup) **Arugula** (Raw 5.0 cal/cup) **Swiss Chard** (Raw, Chopped 6.8 cal/cup) **Spinach** (Raw, Chopped 6.9 cal/cup) **Alfalfa Sprouts** (Raw, 8 cal/cup) **Lettuce** (Iceberg, Raw, Shredded 10.1 cal/cup) **Napa Cabbage** (Cooked 13.1cal/cup) **Cauliflower** (Boiled, Chopped 14.3 cal/cup) **Pickles** (Chopped 16.0 cal/cup) **Cucumber** (Peeled, Raw, Chopped 16.0 cal/cup) **Celery** (Raw, Chopped 16.2 cal/cup) **Okra** (Boiled, Chopped 17.6 cal/cup) **Radishes** (Red, Raw, Chopped 18.6 cal/cup) **Broccoli** (Raw 20.0 cal/cup) **Bok Choy** (Cooked 20.4cal/cup) **Mustard Greens** (Cooked, Chopped 21.0 cal/cup) **New Zealand Spinach** (Boiled 21.6 cal/cup) **Button Mushrooms** (Raw, Chopped 23.5 cal/cup) **Turnip Greens** (Cooked, 27.4 cal/cup) **Zucchini** (Boiled, Chopped 28.8 cal/cup) **Bell Peppers** (Green, Raw, Chopped 29.8 cal/cup) **Leeks** (Boiled, Diced 32.4 cal/cup) **Tomato** (Red, Raw, Chopped 32.4 cal/cup) **Kale** (Raw, Chopped 33.5 cal/cup) **Kelp** (Raw 34 cal/cup) **Turnips** (Boiled, Diced 34.3 cal/cup) **Cabbage** (Boiled, Shredded 34.6 cal/cup) **Eggplant** (Boiled. Diced 35.0 cal/cup) **Figs** (Raw, 37 cal/cup)

This is just a small sampling of the hundreds of foods most of which are readily available and less than 30 calories per ounce. They are all excellent ways to lower your total caloric intake or make room for some of the higher calorie Superfoods that bring high quantities of the Big 43 essential nutrients that your body needs on a daily basis in order to survive and to thrive.

2) EDIBLE RAW PLANTS – Most fruits happen to have far fewer calories than you might suspect. Fruits are good because they; contain no cholesterol, no fat, provide antioxidants and many essential nutrients, and each one brings its own unique array of phytonutrients many of which have already been shown in studies to provide health benefits. Many different fruits and vegetables are featured in the list of Functional Foods in the next chapter because they each bring something significant to the table.

3) LOW GLYCEMIC INDEX FOODS – Even if you aren't diabetic, the low Glycemic Index foods are the way to go. I constantly prattle about "Trash Calories" and now I shall clearly define what this means: 1) Any food high in calories and low in nutritional value: "Nonfunctional Foods" that preclude your chances of eating those Superfoods that are high in calories but also HIGH in NUTRITIONAL VALUE (they are worth it) and 2) Any food high in simple sugars or forms of starch that are easily converted into sugars in the digestive tract and therefore dump a huge amount of sugar into the liver in a very short time. These are the foods with HIGH Glycemic Index values and they irritate the liver and the blood sugar regulatory and metabolic systems. Everyone knows that processed white cane sugar must have a high Glycemic Index and it does: about 103 (higher than straight Glucose because it is a disaccharide – each molecule splits into one Glucose and one Sucrose molecule) but the BIG THREE FOOD CAUSES OF TYPE II DIABETES are just as bad: POTATOES, RICE, and CORN. Once cooked in any way, their starches are converted into forms that are easily broken down into sugars and quickly absorbed and all three have very high Glycemic Index values. Raw bee honey is about 81% sugars and has an average Glycemic Index of about 70. Most preparations of Potatoes, Corn and Rice have GI's that are HIGHER than this. It's not about the AMOUNT of sugars and starches; it is all about the FORMS. Stick to foods with reasonably low Glycemic Index values and very low "Carb Loads;" these are foods that have very little sugar and starch content.

4) LOW FAT FOODS – This one is tricky. While everyone knows that "Whole" milk is high in Saturated Fat, it really only contains 3.25% on average. Since the fats do comprise the bulk of its calories, 1% Skim milk does have about half the calories and is an excellent alternative. Seeds and nuts are the big culprits because even though they are plant foods, they are little solid nuggets of polyunsaturated fats and even though these are the "good kind" they still bring a lot of calories and most seeds and nuts also bring true Saturated Fats as well. But because they are also nutritional powerhouses, they deserve a place in your daily diet, but only in moderation.

5) THE "BIG 43" – Some of these essential nutrients are only present in significant amounts in foods that are high in calories. In order to get everything you need from natural whole foods on a daily basis, the amount of calories those foods would bring would be excessive (well over 2,000 calories per day.) Because of this, you will have to make decisions on which ones you want to get from natural whole foods and which ones you want to take as supplements. Some essential nutrients are only effective when they come from natural foods while others are potentially toxic when they come from supplements; whenever these situations apply, I will point it out.

CONCLUSION

That's a good start towards a "proper diet." Many foods will be explored in great detail in the coming chapters that bring superior health because many are low calorie and excellent sources of the "Big 43" essential nutrients as well as their own unique array of proven beneficial phytonutrients. And it's not all about the plants either, there are Net Negative Calorie meats too and some of them have far better Complete Protein profiles than Beef.

The preceding chapter laid out the foundation for a very effective Natural Whole Foods Diet for achieving and maintaining ideal health, but the cornerstone of success and achieving OPTIMUM THRIVE-LEVEL health rests squarely on being able to get all of the Big 43 essential nutrients in their correct amounts on a daily basis. Although I list the "Top Recommended Supplement" for many of the Big 43 Essential Nutrients:

> I DO NOT ENDORSE ANY PRODUCT. THESE ARE THE BEST I CAN FIND BASED SOLELY ON THE MANUFACTURER'S OWN DESCRIPTIONS WHICH COULD BE MISLEADING.

THE "BIG 43" ESSENTIAL NUTRIENTS

Included is the actual amount of the nutrient needed daily, a brief description of what it does for you, what it does to you when you don't get enough, a comment on the RDA amount if it has been questioned by modern science, the best foods and serving sizes needed to get the proper amount, and the best supplements I have found on the market. I use the term DV – Daily Value, which is usually the RDA amount unless explicitly stated otherwise.

1. VITAMIN A – Plant source Beta-Carotene: 5000IU = 3mg, Animal source Retinol: 5000IU = 1.5mg/day – While Vitamin A is most critical to the human eye, and chronic mild deficiency can lead to poor night vision at first and blindness in severe cases, it is also very important to the skin and chronic deficiency can weaken the skin causing premature aging and making it susceptible not just to wrinkles but also prone to cracking, tearing and infection. Vitamin A is also vital to liver health and chronic deficiency can definitely weaken the liver which handles every molecule of every food you ingest. Current estimates range from 200 to 500 different processes that are performed by the liver all having to do with metabolizing (doing chemistry on) the molecules in our food in order to convert them into suitable forms to pass on to the rest of the body in the bloodstream, regulating those molecules, or building whole new specific molecules for the rest of the body to use. Weakening the liver puts you on a fast track to poor overall health and an early grave.[1]

BETA-CAROTENE (plant source) – BUTTERNUT SQUASH (7.2oz, 457%DV), SWEET POTATO (7oz., 769%DV), CARROTS (raw, chopped, 4.5oz, 428%DV)[1][38][89][136]
RETINOL (animal source) – COD LIVER OIL (1tsp, 90%DV) BEEF LIVER (1oz, 95%DV)[1][47][48]

TOP RECOMMENDED VITAMIN A SUPPLEMENT
==

MANUFACTURER: Any reputable brand
PRODUCT NAME: COD LIVER OIL, 1 Teaspoon/day
A teaspoon of Cod Liver Oil brings 90% of the RDA amount of Vitamin A as the animal form Retinol which is being recommended

by many health professionals in addition to beta-Carotene for OPTIMUM health. A teaspoon of Cod Liver Oil also brings 113% RDA of Vitamin D3, the same one we make in our skin; it also brings about 888mg of the animal Omega-3 fatty acids DHA and EPA which are also required essential nutrients and in this list. [47]

2. VITAMIN B1 – THIAMINE: 1.5mg/day – Thiamine is used by all cells in the body and is involved in energy metabolism and proper liver and brain function. The liver can store excesses for up to 18 days, but because it is a water-soluble vitamin and all cells are hungry for it, it can get used up much faster than that. Thiamine supports skin, eye and digestive tract health and plays a key role in muscle health including and especially the heart. Chronic deficiency of Thiamine can lead to beriberi, a fatal disease. Symptoms of chronic Thiamine deficiency are sundry and nasty including: chronic fatigue, digestive tract issues like colitis or diarrhea, muscle atrophy and weakness, neurological decline including poor memory or confusion, weight loss, poor appetite, nerve damage and inflammation, mood changes like irritability or depression, cardiovascular complications such as enlargement of the heart. [2]

BEST FOOD SOURCES – YEAST EXTRACT SPREAD (1oz, 181%DV), SPIRULINA (3oz, 132%DV), WHEAT GERM (2.5oz, 87%), PORK (lean top loin, 5oz, 60%), PISTACHIOS (3oz, 48%)

Vitamin B1 is difficult but not impossible to get in the 100% RDA amount from natural whole foods. Although processed, Yeast Extract Spread, sold as "Marmite" or "Vegemite," is yeast extract with spices added for flavor and it is extremely nutrient-rich so it doesn't take much to cover Vitamin B1, B2, B3 and B9, and I highly recommend it. Thiamine can be taken in supplement forms, even synthetics which are reportedly safe, however natural extract forms are obviously superior because there is no question about their effectiveness, bioavailability and safety. Extreme overdoses of Thiamine have been shown to be fairly safe but because it does accumulate in the liver, try to stay at or near 100% RDA amount as a daily average.[2][43][56][58][147][151]

3. VITAMIN B2 – RIBOFLAVIN: 1.7mg/day – Riboflavin assists all of the other B Vitamins in energy metabolism and is needed by all cells in the body. It is also believed to be an antioxidant as well. Typical symptoms of Riboflavin deficiency are cracks at the corners of the mouth, sore throat, and sensitivity to bright light. However, Riboflavin plays many critical roles in all cells of the human body and is involved in energy metabolism and protecting DNA from oxidative damage that can lead to cancer. Chronic deficiencies could therefore lead to poor metabolism resulting in chronic fatigue and weakness, obesity, and increase your risk of cancer.[3]

BEST FOOD SOURCES - YEAST EXTRACT SPREAD (1oz, 235%DV), BEEF LIVER (3oz, 135%DV), SPIRULINA (3oz, 181%),

CHICKEN LIVER (3oz, 87%), LAMB (3oz, 50%DV), ALMONDS (3oz, 42%) MILK (whole, 8oz, 26%DV), BUTTON MUSHROOMS (1 cup, 25%DV)[3][31][48][58][74][90][95][116][147]

Without Yeast Extract Spread, sold under the brand names "Marmite" or "Vegemite," Riboflavin is hard to get in 100% RDA amounts on a daily basis. You should look it up and get as much as you can from natural whole foods. One cup of milk and 1 cup of plain white Button Mushrooms will get you about half way there, but after that most other common foods have small amounts in normal portion sizes. Many supplements, especially the B complex products offer Riboflavin in much higher than 100% RDA amounts. Because it is a water soluble vitamin (like all of the B Vitamins) you should try to stay at or near the 100% RDA amount because excesses might get flushed from the body anyway.

4. VITAMIN B3 – NIACIN: 20mg/day – This essential vitamin is also involved in energy metabolism within all cells and chronic deficiency can lead to a disease called Pellagra which is fatal if left unchecked. Symptoms include: dermatitis, digestive difficulties like diarrhea, cognitive decline starting with poor concentration, anxiety and depression and ending in dementia.[4]

BEST FOOD SOURCES – YEAST EXTRACT SPREAD (1oz, 136%DV), TUNA (light, canned in water, 5oz, 83%DV), BEEF SIRLOIN (5oz, 65%DV), CHICKEN (light, w/o skin, w/o bone 4oz, 64%), TURKEY (light, w/o skin, w/o bone 6oz, 60%), PEANUTS (or Peanut butter, 3oz, 57%), SPIRULINA (3oz, 54%), ATLANTIC MACKEREL (4oz, 52%), BEEF LIVER (3oz, 54%), SALMON (4oz, 44%), VEAL (shank, 4oz, 43%), CHICKEN LIVER (3oz, 42%)[4][33][42][48][58][60][61][94][95][141][143][147][149]

Niacin is difficult to get in 100% RDA amounts from natural whole foods without committing to foods high in calories (the peanuts and the sunflower seed kernels are loaded with fats) or cholesterol (the meats.) However, just 1oz. of Yeast Extract Spread, sold as "Marmite" or "Vegemite," brings plenty of Vitamin B1, B2, b3 and B9 and just 44 calories. It has the highest nutrient density of these four very important vitamins that are notoriously difficult to get in sufficient amounts on a daily basis from any other food source. Niacin is a bit unusual amidst the B Vitamins in that most products do not offer over 100% RDA amounts. This is because the actual physical amount of the daily requirement is far larger than the others and because some people experience the "Niacin Flush" when they take it. This is a tingling sensation across the skin. It is not in any way harmful, but it emphasizes the need to around 100% RDA amount daily.

5. VITAMIN B5 – PANTOTHENIC ACID: 10mg/day –

> WATCHOUT – This is a very difficult Vitamin to get in 100% RDA amounts on a Daily basis from Natural Whole Foods.

While deficiency syndrome is rare because most foods contain at least some Pantothenic acid, like all of the other B vitamins it is involved in energy metabolism and brain function. It is also involved in the proper utilization of Vitamin B2, may help reduce LDL (the "bad") cholesterol levels, improve wound healing, and improve digestive tract health. Chronic deficiency can lead to: fatigue, irritability, depression, insomnia, stomach pain, vomiting, upper respiratory infections and burning sensations in the feet.[5]

BEST FOOD SOURCES – SUNFLOWER SEED KERNELS (3oz, 60%DV), BEEF LIVER (3oz, 60%), CHICKEN LIVER (3oz, 51%), AVOCADO (5.3oz, 42%), SALMON (4oz, 37%)[32][42][48][83][95]

Pantothenic acid is found in almost all natural whole foods but in small amounts. Make it a point to look up this Vitamin and make sure you are getting 100%DV on a regular basis.

TOP RECOMMENDED VITAMIN B5 SUPPLEMENT
===

MANUFACTURER: NOW FOODS
PRODUCT NAME: PANTOTHENIC ACID 500MG
WEBSITE: www.nowfoods.com
PRODUCT PAGE: www.nowfoods.com/supplements/
pantothenic-acid-500-mg-capsules

Pantothenic Acid is one of the more difficult B Vitamins to get in 100% RDA amounts from natural whole foods. Rather than take a potentially expensive natural extract source B complex, as long as you take care of B1, B2, B3 and most of the B9 with Yeast Extract Spread, and include some high B9 and B12 foods in your regular diet then you might only need B5, B6, and B7 supplements.

6. VITAMIN B6 – PYRIDOXINE: 2mg/day –

> WATCHOUT – This is a very difficult Vitamin to get in 100% RDA amounts on a Daily basis from Natural Whole Foods.

Vitamin B6 is involved in energy metabolism and brain function like many other B Vitamins but it is also involved in the production of hemoglobin for red blood cells and the regulation of blood sugar. Chronic deficiency syndrome can cause anemia, poor blood sugar regulation, Type II Diabetes, muscle pains, weakness, fatigue, irritability, depression, anxiety, confusion, and increase symptoms of PMS.[6]

BEST FOOD SOURCES – TUNA (light, canned in water, 5oz, 50%DV), PISTACHIOS (3oz, 54%DV), TURKEY (6oz, 50%DV), BANANA (10oz, 52%), BEEF SIRLOIN (5oz, 50%), BEEF LIVER (3oz, 45%), WHEAT GERM (2.5oz, 45%), CHICKEN LIVER (3oz, 36%), SUNFLOWER SEED KERNELS (3oz, 33%), COD (raw 5oz, 30%), SWEET POTATOES (baked w/skin 7oz, 29%)

This is yet another vitamin that slips by unnoticed mainly because we do not need lots of it and deficiency disease is rare because many foods have some B6 in them, but unfortunately it is nowhere near the 100% RDA amount that we should get. This is one of just a few members of the Big 43 that does not have a single natural whole food that can bring 100% of the RDA amount in a reasonable serving size so you need to find a way to make sure you get enough.[43][47][48][56][61][69][95][136][141][149]

TOP RECOMMENDED VITAMIN B6 SUPPLEMENT
==

MANUFACTURER: NOW FOODS
PRODUCT NAME: VITAMIN B-6 50MG TABLETS
WEBSITE: www.nowfoods.com
PRODUCT PAGE: www.nowfoods.com/supplements/
Vitamin-b-6-50mg-tablets

Be aware that this product brings 25 TIMES the Recommended Daily Allowance. However, researchers are finding that some of the established RDA's fall way short of what we actually need on a daily basis. I have found no mention of this regarding Vitamin B6 but very few products offering only Pyridoxine will have less than this amount in them, so you will have to decide for yourself if you want to invest in a dedicated supplement, invest in a complete high quality B Vitamin Complex based on natural extract sources of the vitamins or pursue it in Natural Whole Foods which is the best way to get it, but admittedly very difficult to do.

7. VITAMIN B7 – BIOTIN: 300mcg/day –

WATCHOUT – This is a very difficult Vitamin to get in 100% RDA amounts on a Daily basis from Natural Whole Foods.

While generally thought of as the "beauty vitamin" in that it promotes healthy skin, hair and nails, like all of the B vitamins it plays a role in energy metabolism and brain function as well. Deficiency is very rare because we only need a very small amount daily. The modern consensus is that the average adult actually only needs 30 to 60 mcg (micrograms) not 300mcg recommended by the FDA. And many common foods can cover it easily but, pregnant and nursing mothers may need much more, making it a problem for them. Alcoholics and people with poor liver health are also at risk of Biotin deficiency. Eating a lot of mayonnaise and its kin can lead to Biotin deficiency because mayonnaise and related products like creamy salad dressings and dips are all made from raw eggs which contain Avidin which binds strongly to Biotin and prevents its absorption in the digestive tract. Symptoms of B7 deficiency include: dry irritated skin, brittle hair or hair loss, chronic fatigue, digestive tract issues, muscle aches, nerve damage, mood changes, cramps, tingling in the limbs, and cognitive decline.[7]

BEST FOOD SOURCES – ALMONDS (3oz, 55.78mcg) BEEF LIVER (3oz, about 30mcg) PEANUTS (or Peanut butter, 3oz, 15.31mcg) SWEET POTATO (1 cup. 8.6mcg) ONIONS (1 cup, 8mcg) EGG (1 large, 8mcg) TOMATO (1 cup, 7.2mcg) OATS (½ cup, 7.8mcg) CARROTS (1 cup, 6.1mcg), BANANA (2 lg, 10oz, 6mcg)[7][31][33][38][48][68][69][100][121][136][140]

The biggest problem with Biotin is that it is actually quite difficult to analyze the amount in food. Three different tests are used and sometimes if all three tests are used on a single food, they yield three radically different results. Most people who concentrate on eating a natural whole food diet are expected to get anywhere from 100% to 200%DV (30 to 60mcg daily.)

TOP RECOMMENDED VITAMIN B7 SUPPLEMENT
===

MANUFACTURER: NOW FOODS
PRODUCT NAME: BIOTIN 1000MCG CAPSULES
WEBSITE: www.nowfoods.com
PRODUCT PAGE: www.nowfoods.com/supplements/ biotin-1000-mcg-capsules

This is a huge dose of Biotin and it is a water-soluble vitamin that will likely be eliminated when it is introduced into the body in extreme excess. Also, taking it every few days may not have the desired effect: the body will dump it all on the day you take it and you will be back to no biotin in your body the next day. Therefore it might be worth it to shop around for a product with a lower quantity in it per pill. Many B complex supplements do not even include it, so check the product label and make sure it is in there.

> One last important point: Because VITAMIN B7 – BIOTIN is now believed to have a required DAILY VALUE for dietary intake of 30mcg and not 300mcg, 30mcg is treated as 100%DV – Daily Value – for all discussions in this book.

8. VITAMIN B9 – FOLIC ACID or FOLATE: 400mcg/day – Folate is an exception to the B vitamins in that it does not play a role in energy metabolism but instead assists wit h the copying of the DNA during cell division. It also helps the body use amino acids and Vitamin B12 which is critical to brain function. Symptoms of chronic deficiency include: anemia (poorly formed red blood cells), impaired immune function, poor digestion, and impaired brain function which can include mood changes, memory loss, etc.[8]
BEST FOOD SOURCES – CHICKEN LIVER (3oz, 123%DV), LENTILS (7oz, 90%), MUNG BEANS (7.1oz, 80%), CHICKPEAS (5.8oz, 71%), YEAST EXTRACT SPREAD ("Vegemite" 1oz, 71%), ASPARAGUS (6.3oz, 68%), BEEF LIVER (3oz, 60% DV) WHEAT GERM (2.5oz, 50%DV), SUNFLOWER SEED KERNELS (3oz, 51%DV)[8][32][43][48][63][64][82][95][147][165]

Folate is another B vitamin that is difficult to get unless you plan for it: adding Yeast Extract Spread or a few tablespoons of Wheat Germ to the morning oatmeal greatly helps you to get enough along with many other essential vitamins and minerals.

TOP RECOMMENDED VITAMIN B9 SUPPLEMENT
===

MANUFACTURER: NOW FOODS
PRODUCT NAME: METHYL FOLATE 1000MCG
WEBSITE: www.nowfoods.com
PRODUCT PAGE: www.nowfoods.com/supplements/ methyl-folate-1000-mcg-capsules

Recent studies have shown that a high Folate diet reduces the risk of cancer, but taking Folate supplements does NOT. That should be enough to encourage you to seek out foods high in Folate.

9. VITAMIN B12 – METHYLCOBALAMIN: 6mcg/day –

> WATCHOUT – Most Store-bought B12 products, especially B Vitamin Complex products contain a synthetic form called Cyanocobalamin, that is NOT FOUND IN NATURE.

This is the animal B vitamin, it is almost completely absent from plants and it is of enormous importance for proper brain function. Megadosing with Vitamin B12 has had some limited success in the treatment of Alzheimer's disease and chronic deficiency can lead to: anemia (fewer but larger red blood cells,) balance and walking difficulties, nerve damage, confusion, muscle atrophy, loss of the ability to sense vibration, and dementia. [9]

BEST FOOD SOURCES - CLAMS (1oz, 461%DV), BEEF LIVER (1oz, 277%DV), SARDINES (2.5oz, 100%DV) [9][48][54][62]

Vitamin B12 has the smallest RDA amount of any nutrient in this list but it has the highest importance because it is the "Brain Vitamin." As such plants don't make it, so it has to come from animal foods. The synthetic form found in almost all store-bought supplements is called Cyanocobalamin which is different from the one found in the human brain and should be avoided.

TOP RECOMMENDED VITAMIN B12 SUPPLEMENT
==

MANUFACTURER: NOW FOODS
PRODUCT NAME: METHYL B-12 1000MCG LOZENGES
WEBSITE: www.nowfoods.com
PRODUCT PAGE: www.nowfoods.com/supplements/ Methyl-b-12-1000-mcg-lozenges

Don't be too alarmed about the amount of Vitamin B12 in each of these pills, studies are starting to show that we can use far more of the B vitamins on a daily basis than what the FDA recommends. This quality product from a quality vendor provides it in the correct form: Methylcobalamin from a non-animal based source.

VITAMIN B COMPLEX

Don't ignore the B vitamins. Every one of them is involved in BRAIN FUNCTION and the brain is "you-the-person." So when it is not working right, then you-the-person aren't working right either. A shortage of any one of these critical nutrients can start to mess with your MENTAL STATE and bring on such things as anxiety, depression, confusion and even memory loss. I don't advocate multivitamins, but I do RECOMMEND B Vitamin supplements including a B Complex if you feel that you cannot track them all down on a daily basis. Store-bought products contain nothing but synthetic versions and there are many health professionals who are unconvinced of the effectiveness and safety of these forms. There are only a few Vitamin B Complex supplements from specialty vendors that contain naturally extracted B vitamins.

Some are not complete (don't contain all eight B vitamins in at least 100% RDA amounts) and others are extremely high priced and likely not worth the money.

TOP RECOMMENDED VITAMIN B COMPLEX SUPPLEMENT
===

MANUFACTURER: Garden of Life
PRODUCT NAME: VITAMIN CODE – RAW B COMPLEX
WEBSITE: www.gardenoflife.com
PRODUCT PAGE: www.gardenoflife.com/content/product/
vitamin-code-raw-b-complex/

This is the most complete Vitamin B Complex supplement that I have been able to find and all eight of the B vitamins (including Biotin which is often left out of B Complex supplements) are included in better than 100% RDA amounts and all of them are extracted from natural sources. It is not inexpensive, but it is by far the highest quality B Complex I could find and for the price it is actually a very good deal; you get them all in natural forms and plenty of peace of mind that you have them all 100% covered.

10. VITAMIN C – L-ASCORBIC ACID: 60mg/day – Vitamin C plays many roles in all cells in the human body and it is also an antioxidant. Extreme deficiency can lead to a disease called Scurvy which is fatal. Chronic deficiency symptoms include: easy bruising, swollen, bleeding or inflamed gums, slow wound healing, dry and splitting hair, dry red spots on the skin, rough, dry, scaly skin, nose bleeds, impaired immune system, digestive tract problems, slowed metabolism, and swollen painful joints. One reliable source also indicates that chronic deficiency can lead to: gallbladder disease, stroke, cancer, high blood pressure and atherosclerosis. [11]

BEST FOOD SOURCES – GUAVA (5.8oz, 628%DV), KIWI (6.25oz, 273%DV), GRAPEFRUIT (9oz, 135%), CABBAGE (4oz, 100%DV)[11][35][36][37][163]

I always prefer the natural whole foods first, after that I only recommend supplements made from natural extracts. In many cases these products are so expensive that it is literally more economical to just buy and eat the fruits (or cabbage.)

BEST VITAMIN C SUPPLEMENTS
===

MANUFACTURER: NATURE'S WAY
PRODUCT NAME: ALIVE! VITAMIN C POWDER
WEBSITE: www.naturesway.com
PRODUCT PAGE: www.naturesway.com/Product-
Catalog/Alive-Vitamin-C-Powder-120-grams
===

MANUFACTURER: RADIANT LIFE
PRODUCT NAME: PURE SYNERGY PURE RADIANCE C
WEBSITE: www.radiantlifecatalog.com

PRODUCT PAGE: www.radiantlifecatalog.com/product/pure-radiance-c/

You can take plain old store bought Vitamin C, but it is synthetic and there are many health professionals saying that it is potentially TOXIC while others insist that it is safe. Vitamin C (L-Ascorbic Acid) is water soluble, but eating the fruit provides a lot more than just the juices. (Buy 100% natural juices; not ENRICHED ones.)

11. VITAMIN D3 – CHOLECALCIFEROL: 400IU = 10mcg/day – A recent study determined that around 42% of the U.S. population is chronically deficient in Vitamin D3. An irony since it is one of the few vitamins that we can make ourselves, but it does require about two 20 minute exposures of the face and arms to direct sunlight without sunscreen for this to happen. Vitamin D3 is directly linked to the body's ability to utilize Calcium, but it has many more roles than that and deficiency symptoms include: weakness, chronic fatigue, depression, insomnia, anxiety, weak bones, impaired immune system, inflammation and swelling. Since Calcium is needed by the cardiovascular system for blood vessel construction and maintenance and also by the brain, Vitamin D3 deficiency can lead to diminished brain function, as well as cardiovascular disease which is a contributing factor of high blood pressure and fatal complications (like heart attack.)[12]

BEST FOOD SOURCES – SALMON (wild, 4oz, 148%DV), COD LIVER OIL (1tsp, 113%DV), ATLANTIC MACKEREL (4oz, 100%), SARDINES (4oz, 76%), MILK (8oz, 24%DV) [42][47][60][62][116]

The best way to get all of the Vitamin D3 that you need is with two 20 minute exposures to direct sunlight. After that only fish can bring enough to satisfy the RDA of this critical vitamin.

TOP RECOMMENDED VITAMIN D3 SUPPLEMENT
===

MANUFACTURER: Any reputable brand

PRODUCT NAME: COD LIVER OIL, 1 Tsp/day

One teaspoon brings 90% Vitamin A as Retinol (the preferred form) as well as 113% Vitamin D3 and 888mg of the Omega-3 fatty acids DHA and EPA which are essential nutrients needed for cardiovascular health. DO NOT EXCEED 100% RDA DAILY.

12. VITAMIN E – TOCOPHEROLS AND TOCOTRIENOLS: 30 IU/day = 20mg as d-alpha-Tocopherol – I believe that Vitamin E deficiency is rampant in the U.S. because most people do not eat a lot of seeds and nuts which are the primary source of this crucial vitamin. Vitamin E actually occurs in about 8 different molecular forms and while most people believe that it is the "Energy vitamin" it is actually a very powerful antioxidant and is involved in proper immune function, brain function, proper blood clotting, promotes healthy skin and hair, promotes eye health and participates in proper gene expression. Chronic deficiency results in: muscle pain, weakness, vision problems, numbness, impaired immune system, loss of balance, tremors, and difficulty walking. Because

Vitamin E is needed for proper blood clotting, chronic deficiency could very well increase your risk of heart attack or stroke. [13]

BEST FOOD SOURCES – SUNFLOWER SEED KERNELS (3oz, 111%DV), ALMONDS (3oz, 108%DV), PEANUTS (and Peanut butter, 3oz, 39%DV)[31][32][33]

Vitamin E is incredibly important for overall health and participates in the protection of the DNA in all cells making it a safety blanket against cancer and chronic deficiency may be a significant risk factor contributing to the rising rates of cancer worldwide. Vitamin E is OIL SOLUBLE; it is difficult for the body to handle: DO NOT EXCEED 100% RDA daily.

TOP RECOMMENDED VITAMIN E SUPPLEMENTS
==

MANUFACTURER: JARROW FORMULAS
PRODUCT NAME: FAMIL-E
WEBSITE: www.jarrow.com
PRODUCT PAGE: www.jarrow.com/product/292/Famil-E
==

MANUFACTURER: NOW FOODS
PRODUCT NAME: VITAMIN E 200 IU MIXED
        TOCOPHEROLS SOFTGELS
WEBSITE: www.nowfoods.com
PRODUCT PAGE: www.nowfoods.com/supplements/vitamin-e-200-iu-mixed-tocopherols-softgels
==

MANUFACTURER: Dr. MERCOLA
PRODUCT NAME: MERCOLA VITAMIN E
WEBSITE: www.mercola.com
PRODUCT PAGE: https://products.mercola.com/vitamine/
These three products include many forms of Vitamin E and are recommended for those trying to avoid seeds and nuts. There is evidence that CHRONIC EXCESS MAY CAUSE STROKE.

13. VITAMIN K – PHYLLOQUINONE -K1, MENAQUINONE -K2: 80mcg/day – Vitamin K plays a vital role in bone metabolism, the proper utilization of Calcium by the body, proper blood clotting and proper blood sugar regulation. Symptoms of deficiency include but are certainly not limited to: easy bruising, excessive bleeding, tooth decay and weakened bones. Because of the critical role it plays in the maintenance of blood vessels and bones, deficiency is a likely contributing factor of atherosclerosis, arteriosclerosis, hypertension, and osteoporosis. [14]

BEST FOOD SOURCES – COLLARD GREENS (boiled, 6.7oz, 1045%), SWISS CHARD (raw, 6.2oz, 636%), KALE (raw, 1.2oz, 347%), BROCCOLI (5.5oz, 245%), BRUSSELS SPROUTS (5.5oz, 243%), CABBAGE (5.3oz, 204%) SPINACH (1.1oz, 181%), ASPARAGUS (6.3oz, 114%) [14][37][49][66][67][82][87][98][137]

Kale is even higher in Vitamin K1 than Spinach, but Collards blow everything else away. Dried Plums are an excellent source of

Vitamin K as well. Most people believe that Vitamin K will lead to internal blood clotting and avoid it which is a tragic irony since Vitamin K actually promotes PROPER blood clotting and chronic deficiency can lead to internal blood clotting which can kill. Be sure to get it from these inexpensive low calorie natural foods.

TOP RECOMMENDED VITAMIN K SUPPLEMENT
==

MANUFACTURER: NOW FOODS
PRODUCT NAME: VITAMIN K2 100MCG VEG CAPSULES
WEBSITE: www.nowfoods.com
PRODUCT PAGE: www.nowfoods.com/supplements/vitamin-k-2-100-mcg-veg-capsules

Vitamin K is too easy to get from natural whole foods like Spinach and Kale which are highly recommended. Vitamin K is another OIL SOLUBLE VITAMIN: DO NOT EXCEED 100% RDA AMOUNTS DAY AFTER DAY. Be sure it is NOT SYNTHETIC. ALL synthetic forms of Vitamin K (K3, K4, and K5) are TOXIC.

14. CALCIUM: 1000mg/day – We all know the bones and teeth are made out of Calcium compounds, but it plays other daily critical roles and does get used up and tossed out on a daily basis. Just because you have stopped growing doesn't mean that you no longer need Calcium. In fact, the bones are designed specifically to be able to dissolve the Calcium and release it back into the blood on a daily basis and the bones get recycled about once every ten years because of this process. Calcium supports balancing blood pH, is used in the continual maintenance of blood vessel walls, is used in nerve communication, and is involved in brain chemistry. We go through about 1000mg of Calcium each day and chronic dietary deficiency will erode the bones as they try to keep up with that demand. Symptoms include: higher chance of developing osteopenia or osteoporosis, tooth decay, weak bones, fractures, muscle tension, high blood pressure, arteriosclerosis, inflammation, increased severity of PMS symptoms, indigestion, higher risk for kidney and gall stones (an irony since these are made out of calcium compounds,) higher risk for heart disease, higher risk of diabetes and higher risk for cancer.[15]

BEST FOOD SOURCES – PARMESAN/ROMANO CHEESE (3oz, 100%DV), SWISS CHEESE (3oz, 66%DV), YOGURT (8oz, 30%DV), MILK (8oz, 30%DV) [15][44][45][46][116]

Not only do we need a large amount of Calcium daily but we also need proper amounts of Vitamin D3, Vitamin K, Chromium, Magnesium, and Lysine so the body can properly use all of that Calcium.

TOP RECOMMENDED CALCIUM SUPPLEMENT
==

MANUFACTURER: NOW FOODS
PRODUCT NAME: CALCIUM CITRATE VEG CAPSULES
WEBSITE: www.nowfoods.com

If you are going to take the Calcium, then you must also make absolutely certain that you are also getting at least 100% RDA amounts of Chromium, Magnesium, Vitamin D3, and Vitamin K. Lysine is an essential amino acid that is also required, but you will get enough from 100% amount of Complete Protein, covered further down and it is relatively easy to resolve.

15. CHLORINE: 2500mg/day – This unusual requirement, a toxin to most life forms on Earth, is required in significant amounts for use in some specialized nerve pathways (functioning as an electrolyte) and is also used by most tissues to support proper osmotic function (the movement of nutrients into the cells and waste by-products out of them) and for the hydrochloric acid in the stomach. Deficiency syndrome is almost unheard of because most people get enough salt to suffice.[154]

BEST FOOD SOURCES – IODIZED OR SEA SALT (½ tsp/day)

Make certain that you do not overdo it with salt. Excessive Sodium levels in the blood are terrible for your health and cause high blood pressure. Watch the Salt content of packaged foods. Two MAJOR culprits of dumping far too much poor quality salt in them (no iodine) are canned soup and frozen pizza.

16. CHOLINE: 550mg/day –

> WATCHOUT – This is a VERY difficult essential nutrient to get in the 100% RDA amount from Natural Whole Foods.

Deficiency syndrome of Choline is prevalent. One of the major problems associated with this nutrient is that different people have significantly different requirements for it. It is estimated that 50% of the population have genes that create a higher methyl metabolism and since Choline is involved in these processes this can lead to a higher requirement for it and thus a higher likelihood of deficiency. Choline is also difficult to absorb in the digestive tract and chronic liver problems can also lead to severe deficiency. Some forms also have difficulty in crossing the blood-brain barrier as well. Choline is related in molecular structure to the B vitamins and deficiency symptoms are similar and include: low energy levels, fatigue, memory loss, cognitive decline, learning disabilities, muscle aches, nerve damage, mood changes and possibly other psychological problems. The best forms are Alpha- Glycerylphosphorylcholine a.k.a. Alpha-GPC and Citicholine.[10]

BEST FOOD SOURCES – BEEF LIVER (3oz. 50%DV), CHICKEN LIVER (3oz, 30%), SHRIMP (4oz, 36%DV), SALMON (6 oz, 50%DV), EGGS (1 large, 25%DV)[10][42][48][95][100][132]

This is a very difficult nutrient to get in 100% RDA amounts daily because we need a relatively large amount of it and many people have vastly different requirements for it and there are many chronic conditions that can inhibit its absorption and utilization by the body even when it is plentiful in the natural foods they eat.

TOP RECOMMENDED CHOLINE SUPPLEMENTS

==

MANUFACTURER: NOW FOODS
PRODUCT NAME: CHOLINE & INOSITOL, 500 MG, 100 CAPSULES
WEBSITE: www.nowfoods.com
PRODUCT PAGE: www.nowfoods.com/supplements/choline-inositol-500-mg-capsules

==

MANUFACTURER: NOW FOODS
PRODUCT NAME: ALPHA GPC, 300 MG, 60 CAPSULES
WEBSITE: www.nowfoods.com
PRODUCT PAGE: www.nowfoods.com/supplements/alpha-gpc-300-mg-veg-capsules

These products from a quality vendor come highly recommended. The first also provides Inositol, another nutrient related to Choline which many professionals are beginning to indicate is a required essential nutrient as well. And the second contains the form Alpha-GPC which has been proven to be able to pass across the blood-brain barrier and is therefore a superior form. I recommend both and don't scrimp on the Alpha-GPC which is expensive from any vendor, but gives the brain cells this critical nutrient they need to create their neurotransmitters and is too important to ignore.

17. CHROMIUM: 120mcg/day –

WATCHOUT – This is a very difficult mineral to get in the 100% RDA amount from most Natural Whole Foods.

This one is HUGE in terms of what it does for us, it plays countless critical roles in cellular metabolism throughout all cells in the body and we only need it in micrograms, but deficiency does occur because it is hard to find in sufficient quantities in most foods. And deficiency can have dire consequences: poor blood glucose regulation, weak bones and bone loss, low energy, fatigue, degradation of the skin, higher risk for high cholesterol and heart disease, poor concentration and memory, deterioration of eye health, mood changes like anxiety, changes in appetite, changes in weight, stunted growth and development, delayed time in healing wounds or recovering from surgery. The contribution to bone loss is a key factor. It means that the bones are releasing too much calcium into the blood which can and will manifest itself as osteoporosis or other serious bone disease as well as pose a threat for cardiovascular disease including atherosclerosis which can cause or exacerbate high blood pressure although long term deficiency leads directly to Type II "late onset" Diabetes and is the primary concern.[17]

BEST FOOD SOURCES – BROCCOLI (boiled, 5.5oz, 53%DV), GRAPE JUICE (100% PURE CONCORD, 8oz, 32%DV), GARLIC (1tsp fresh minced, 12%DV)[17][49][50][51]

About 2 cups of Broccoli or 24 oz. of 100% Concord Grape Juice (or similar dark grape juice) can bring you the 100% RDA amount. Chromium participates in insulin pathways and helps the body regulate blood sugar levels and use sugars properly. Chronic deficiency is likely the #1 cause of Type II Diabetes worldwide.

TOP RECOMMENDED CHROMIUM SUPPLEMENT

==

MANUFACTURER: JARROW FORMULAS
PRODUCT NAME: CHROMIUM GTF, 200 MCG, 100 CAPS
WEBSITE: www.jarrow.com
PRODUCT PAGE: www.jarrow.com/product/214/Chromium_ GTF

This product provides Chromium in fermented yeast rather than Chromium picolinate which is being questioned by the medical industry concerning its effectiveness and safety. The RDA is 120mcg (micrograms) which may be anywhere from 2 to 4 times what most studies and health professionals have determined that the average adult actually needs. As such, this product should be taken no more than once every other day although once every three to five days would be OK. That will help offset the expense.

18. COPPER: 2mg/day – Copper is found in at least seven enzymes involved in energy metabolism reactions. We do not need a lot of it, but it is necessary for proper health and severe chronic deficiency although very rare, could be life-threatening. It is also involved in the construction of the sulfur based amino acids used in all proteins and especially the joints. Deficiency syndrome results in: low energy, fatigue, and painful and inflamed joints. Chronic excess can lead to copper poisoning which is dangerous and difficult to fix.[18]

BEST FOOD SOURCES – OYSTERS (1oz, 62%DV) CLAMS (2.5oz, 25%DV) BEEF LIVER (3oz, 400%DV) WALNUTS (2oz, 44%DV) ALMONDS (3oz, 48%) SUNFLOWER SEED KERNELS (3oz, 78%) PUMPKIN SEEDS (5oz, 50%DV) DARK CHOCOLATE (4oz, 180%DV) PISTACHIOS (3oz, 57%DV) PEANUTS (3oz, 21%DV) SPIRULINA (3oz, 255%DV)

Many superfoods bring copper and some bring it in excessive quantities. Most seeds and nuts will cover your RDA easily but try not to exceed the 100% RDA amount daily over long periods because in chronic excessive amounts Copper, like most minerals, can become TOXIC. [18][30][31][32][33][48][53][54][55][56][57][58]

TOP RECOMMENDED COPPER SUPPLEMENT

==

MANUFACTURER: SOLGAR
PRODUCT NAME: CHELATED COPPER, 100 TABLETS
WEBSITE: www.solgar.com

Solgar products can be found at many major online supplement retailers. The manufacturer also notes that Copper is involved in the formation of collagen and connective tissues supporting the skin, bones and joints. Excesses of Copper can become TOXIC with potentially severe adverse reactions and even though this product is a chelated form, you should only take Copper if you are certain that your diet has very little if any Copper in it. The Natural Whole Foods Diet does have many foods very high in Copper, so check the foods you regularly eat online at nutritiondata.self.com to be sure you are not drastically exceeding what you need day after day. To be clear: most people eating a well balanced natural whole foods diet DO NOT NEED TO TAKE COPPER.

19. IODINE: 150mcg/day – Iodine is in the hormones made by the thyroid. Deficiency was eliminated for fifty years until the medical industry went on their Anti-Sodium/Anti-Salt crusade starting in the late 1970's. Now deficiency is on the rise because people have sworn off salt, specifically Iodized Salt, so where are you getting your Iodine? Underactive thyroid messes with your body's overall metabolism and can have severe long term consequences: trouble producing saliva and properly digesting food, swollen salivary glands and dry mouth, skin problems, poor concentration and short term memory loss, muscle pains and weakness, increased risk for thyroid disease, increased risk for fibrosis and fibromyalgia. Estimates are that 50% of the world's population is suffering from chronic Iodine deficiency and I believe this results in underactive thyroid which is the leading cause of obesity and the DESIRE to stay inactive because of the severely reduced metabolism and resulting fatigue.[19]

BEST FOOD SOURCES – IODIZED SALT (½ tsp, 100%DV), SEA SALT (½ tsp, 100%DV), KELP (dried, 1 sheet, 10% to 2000%), COD (Wild, 4.5oz, 100%DV), YOGURT (8oz, 47%). EGGS (1 large, 16%DV) [19][46][72][96][100]

As long as you have dropped all of the fast food, junk food, packaged, processed and canned foods laced with POOR QUALITY salt with no Iodine in it, you can now go back to consuming about ½ teaspoon of IODIZED SALT per day; SEA SALT is said to contain a better form and either salt is the easiest way to get your necessary Iodine. For those who need to stay away from salt altogether, all supplements are Potassium Iodide which is as safe as Iodized salt. Do not exceed 100% RDA daily because excesses in Iodine can also lead to Thyroid malfunction and disease which is very serious and easily avoided.[19]

20. IRON: 18mg/day –

WATCHOUT – Unless you are paying attention to this critical mineral, you are very likely suffering from chronic deficiency which can be life-threatening.

We all know that Iron is used to make hemoglobin and that deficiency will lead to anemia, but did you know that it is also used in all muscle cells in a compound called myoglobin? This is the molecule that takes the oxygen away from the hemoglobin in the blood. The World Health Organization estimates that 80% of the world's population is chronically deficient in Iron. That includes the beef-eating U.S. because even liver, a food source from the cow with a high concentration of Iron, would take 3/4 POUND a day to provide enough and no one eats that much. Chronic deficiency symptoms are myriad and potentially life threatening: fatigue, weakness, pale skin, shortness of breath, dizziness, cravings to eat items that aren't food, such as dirt, ice or clay, tingling or crawling feeling in the legs, swollen or sore tongue, cold hands and feet, fast or irregular heartbeat, brittle nails, inability to focus or concentrate, headaches, weakened immune system, and digestive problems including Irritable Bowel Syndrome. Iron deficiency can affect the HEART and deficiency can play a contributing factor to not just cardiac disease but heart failure as well.[20]

BEST FOOD SOURCES – CLAMS (canned, 2.5oz, 100%DV), SPIRULINA (dried, 3oz, 132%DV), DARK CHOCOLATE (100% pure, 4oz, 100%DV), CHICKEN LIVER (3oz, 42%), LENTILS (7oz, 37%), CHICKPEAS (5.8oz, 26%), BLACK BEANS (8.5oz, 25%), BEEF LIVER (3oz, 24%DV), SWISS CHARD (6.2oz, 22%)

Very few foods have enough Iron in them to meet our 100% requirements of this critical mineral so be sure you get enough daily. Three of the craziest foods have enough: canned Clams, Spirulina and Dark Chocolate.[39][48][54][57][58][63][64][95][137]

TOP RECOMMENDED IRON SUPPLEMENT
==

MANUFACTURER: SOLGAR
PRODUCT NAME: GENTLE IRON, 25 MG, 180 VEGETABLE CAPSULES
WEBSITE: www.solgar.com
This product provides Iron in the chelated form Iron Bisglycinate which is gentler on the stomach according to the manufacturer and does not cause constipation like most other forms do. 25mg is 139% RDA so this product is also providing a very good dose of this critical mineral. Do NOT overdo it with Iron. The liver absorbs a lot of it for its own use in all of its sundry activities and taking too much IN SUPPLEMENTS will definitely lead to Iron POISONING which is disastrous for your liver and could end up being DEADLY.

21. MAGNESIUM: 400mg/day –

> WATCHOUT – We need a LOT of this mineral on a daily basis and most people are not getting nearly enough which can be disastrous to your health.

This mineral plays numerous roles in cellular metabolism ranging from the proper regulation of blood sugar to the proper utilization of Calcium. It is also a significant blood serum electrolyte. It is also needed for the body to properly utilize Calcium. Chronic deficiency has been linked to causing: Alzheimer's disease, Type II Diabetes, increased insulin resistance, cardiovascular disease, migraines, hypertension, ADHD, and heart disease.[21]

BEST FOOD SOURCES – DARK CHOCOLATE (100% pure, 4oz,

92%DV), PUMPKIN SEEDS (4oz, 72%DV), ALMONDS (3oz, 60%DV), CASHEWS (3oz, 59%DV), SPIRULINA (dried, 3oz, 42%), WHEAT GERM (2.5oz, 42%), SWISS CHARD (6.2oz, 36%), PEANUTS (3oz, 33%) [21][31][33][43][61][62][55][57][58][92][137]

Getting enough Magnesium daily can be a real challenge but we do need a LOT of it so you must pay attention to it and all of the minerals which are categorically difficult to get in 100% RDA amounts daily. By the way, 100% Pure Dark Chocolate brings 100%DV of Iron AND Magnesium and that's why it is a Top Recommended Superfood. Unfortunately, it also brings over 600 calories and too much Copper so you cannot depend on it daily and you will have to piece together Magnesium from other foods.

TOP RECOMMENDED MAGNESIUM SUPPLEMENT
===
MANUFACTURER: NOW FOODS
PRODUCT NAME: MAGNESIUM CITRATE, 120 VEG CAPSULES
WEBSITE: www.nowfoods.com
PRODUCT PAGE: www.nowfoods.com/supplements/ magnesium-citrate-veg-capsules

Magnesium Citrate is a chelated form. Chelate simply means a molecular bonding structure that breaks down slowly, so it won't be completely broken down in the stomach, but is also high in bioavailability in the intestines. You can find this compound as a liquid laxative, but most products advise taking the entire 8 to 10 oz. bottle which will act like a strong laxative. In this form most products contain 200 mg of actual Magnesium per ounce. One to two tablespoons in the morning and again in the evening should work, but it could still make your bowels "loose" so try this on a weekend! By the way, there is no guarantee that the capsules will not act as a laxative as well. Two other unusual sources that I have seen some health professionals supporting are Milk of Magnesia and Epsom salt. It should be clear that products bringing concentrated forms of Magnesium in them have significant effects on our digestive tract. Milk of Magnesia's active ingredient is Magnesium Hydroxide (MgOH,) a strong alkaline that reacts with stomach acid neutralizing it and resulting in water and Magnesium Chloride which is highly soluble and the digestive tract will be able to absorb the Magnesium in this form. Magnesium makes up about 56% of the Magnesium Hydroxide molecule (it is a very light metal) and one teaspoon of a typical product claims to contain 400mg of MgOH. That's roughly 224mg of Magnesium. One teaspoon an hour or two after breakfast and one in the afternoon between lunch and dinner (taking too much at once can act like a laxative as well) will bring you the daily requirement of this critical mineral. Epsom salt (Magnesium Sulfate) is a powerful laxative and I personally do not recommend it although, like the other Magnesium products, the digestive tract can absorb the Magnesium in this form.

22. MANGANESE: 2mg/day –Manganese is only needed in small quantities, but it participates in numerous critical roles including: proper enzyme function, nutrient absorption, wound healing, and bone development. Deficiency syndrome is rare, but since it is involved in nutrient absorption, deficiency can result in any number of random deficiency symptoms caused by a lack of any of the other nutrients.[22]

BEST FOOD SOURCES – CLAMS (canned, 2.5oz, 35%DV), WALNUTS (2oz, 96%DV), ALMONDS (3oz, 111%DV), SUNFLOWER SEED KERNELS (3oz, 90%DV), PISTACHIOS (3oz, 54%DV) CHICKPEAS (5oz, 70%DV) OATS (2oz, 100%DV) BANANAS (10oz, 40%DV) DARK CHOCOLATE (4oz, 232%DV) SPIRULINA (3oz, 81%DV)

Many superfoods like seeds, nuts, and oatmeal are LOADED with Manganese and if you are switching to them you will certainly get your fill. Extreme excesses of Manganese (and most of the other minerals as well) can be TOXIC. So be careful of the foods you choose and try to stay near the 100% RDA amount as a weekly average and do not exceed the 100% RDA amount day after day.[22][30][31][32][54][56][58][63][68][69]

TOP RECOMMENDED MANGANESE SUPPLEMENT
==
MANUFACTURER: BLUEBONNET NUTRITION
PRODUCT NAME: CHELATED MANGANESE, 90 VCAPS
WEBSITE: www.bluebonnetnutrition.com
PRODUCT: bluebonnetnutrition.com/product/118/
Albion%AE_Chelated_Manganese_Vcaps

Only take this supplement after you check your regular dietary foods at nutritiondata.self.com to establish that you are not getting enough. Under normal circumstances anyone eating a well varied natural foods diet WILL NOT NEED TO TAKE A MANGANESE SUPPLEMENT.

23. MOLYBDENUM: 75mcg/day – Although only needed in very trace amounts, Molybdenum plays a key role in sulfur metabolism. Without it our body cannot use the sulfur in our foods and cannot build its own sulfur based compounds which include: Vitamin B1 – Thiamine and several amino acids involved in all proteins in all cells in the body and in particular the proteins including collagen used in ligaments, tendons, skin, hair and nails. Severe deficiency in infants can be life threatening and it is also serious trouble for adults.[23]

BEST FOOD SOURCES – LENTILS (7oz, 330%), LIMA BEANS (8.5oz, 300%), BLACK BEANS (8.5oz, 275%DV), CHICKPEAS (5.8oz, 273%), GREEN PEAS (canned 6oz, 192%), OATS (1.4oz, precooked, 64%)[23][39][63][64][68][70][112]

Eating two servings of any of these foods during the week will ensure that you are getting plenty of Molybdenum; the seeds of many fast growing plants are loaded with it. As with all of the minerals, do not exceed the 100% RDA by drastic amounts over a long period because it can become TOXIC.

TOP RECOMMENDED MOLYBDENUM SUPPLEMENT
==

MANUFACTURER: COUNTRY LIFE
PRODUCT NAME: CHELATED MOLYBDENUM, 150 MCG, 100 TABLETS
WEBSITE: www.countrylifevitamins.com
PRODUCT: www.countrylifevitamins.com/store/chelated-
molybdenum-150-mcg,

If you are eating the legumes and Oats regularly, chances are you do not need this supplement. If you do decide to take it, the pills contain double the RDA amount and unless your doctor has prescribed it, just one capsule every other day should suffice.

24. PHOSPHORUS: 1000mg/day –

WATCHOUT – Excessive intake of Phosphorus can place a terrible strain on your kidneys. CAUTION IS ADVISED.

The bones are made from Calcium Phosphate structures and Phosphorus is also found in several amino acids and provides the cross-links in every DNA molecule. No phosphorus means no new proteins or DNA can be made so no new cells can be built and grow which halts the ongoing renewal process of virtually all organ systems. Phosphorus is common in all foods and deficiency is very rare, but possible if a person is not adhering to a natural whole food diet and symptoms include: weak bones, osteoporosis, changes in appetite, joint pain, muscle aches, difficulty exercising, tooth decay, numbness and tingling, rapid weight loss or gain, stunted growth, developmental problems, poor concentration or anxiety.[24]

BEST FOOD SOURCES – SUNFLOWER SEED KERNELS (3oz, 96%DV), PEANUTS (and Peanut butter, 3oz, 30%DV), DARK CHOCOLATE (100% pure,, 4oz, 44%DV), PISTACHIOS (3oz, 42%DV), BRAZIL NUTS (1oz, 20%DV), SWISS CHEESE (3oz, 48%DV), PARMESAN/ROMANO CHEESE (3 oz, 60%DV) MILK (8oz, 22%DV) [24][32][33][44][45][56][57][65][116]

Most foods contain Phosphorus but we do need a lot of it (1000mg/day.) Phosphorus has been linked to detoxification of the body and this is part of the reason that it causes trouble for the kidneys. Folks with kidney problems are advised to stay on a low Phosphorus diet and if you suspect that you have weak kidneys you should check with a doctor before pursuing Phosphorus. I DO NOT RECOMMEND PHOSPHORUS SUPPLEMENTS because they can be very harsh on the kidneys.

TOP RECOMMENDED PHOSPHORUS SUPPLEMENT
==

MANUFACTURER: NOW FOODS
PRODUCT NAME: BONE MEAL
WEBSITE: www.nowfoods.com

Since most foods contain Phosphorus, anyone eating an average amount of any food daily should get enough to fulfill their needs. Our digestive tracts are very good at absorbing Phosphorus in Phosphate form which is added to many different packaged foods, but virtually all natural foods are high in Phosphorus in good natural forms. For the elderly who do not have a history of kidney trouble, I do recommend taking Calcium in the form of Calcium Phosphate (Bone Meal) because other products like Calcium carbonate (a.k.a. limestone) or Calcium citrate tend to block the absorption of Phosphorus, and their diets are usually not adequate to supply enough of either Calcium or Phosphorus. However, the cautions remain: you must also get at least 100% RDA amounts of Vitamin D3, Vitamin K, Magnesium, Chromium, Manganese and Lysine (an amino acid found in Complete Protein) in order for the body to properly utilize all of that Calcium otherwise you are just building Kidney and Gall bladder stones with those supplements.

25. POTASSIUM: 3500mg/day –

> WATCHOUT – Potassium has the highest requirement of any vitamin or mineral and NO ONE is getting what they need on a daily basis.
>
> GRADUALLY increase your daily intake of this critical mineral because it can put a terrible strain on the kidneys so CAUTION IS ADVISED.

This is the BIG one. The FDA recently increased the RDA of Potassium from 3200mg per day to 3500mg. It is the single largest quantity of any essential nutrient in the Big 43 list (other than a few of the essential amino acids) and it amounts to about one heaping teaspoon of Potassium Chloride. NO ONE is getting enough Potassium from a natural whole food diet because even the foods with the highest amounts, Avocados and Bananas, do not have enough to satisfy our large requirement for this critical mineral. It would take THREE average sized avocados and I have trouble eating ONE and that would also bring THOUSANDS of calories. It takes EIGHT large bananas which would also bring nearly a thousand calories although that would also bring 100% RDA of much needed Dietary Fiber as well. Potassium is involved in the synapses between the nerve endings and the muscle cells (along with Sodium) and chronic deficiency can lead to acute deficiency resulting in rapid involuntary muscle twitching and there is ONE muscle in which this should never happen: your HEART (can result in palpitations and heart attack.) Potassium plays a critical role in maintaining proper fluid balance and blood pressure and chronic deficiency might be the leading cause of high blood pressure primarily because it is so difficult to get enough daily. Other symptoms of Potassium deficiency (hypokalemia) can include: migraines, dehydration, swelling of glands and tissues, fatigue, constipation, muscle cramps, weight gain, cellulite buildup, nausea, arthritis, bloating, irritability, depression, confusion, even hallucinations.[25]

BEST FOOD SOURCES – DRIED PLUMS (6.1oz, 36%DV), SPIRULINA (dried, 3oz, 33%), SWEET POTATO (baked w/skin, 7oz, 27%), LOW SODIUM ORIGINAL V-8 VEGETABLE JUICE (8oz, 23%DV), BANANA (1 large, 14%DV) [58][69][73][136][157]

Potassium is another potential problem for weak kidneys and you should check your kidney health with your doctor before GRADUALLY ramping up your daily dosage to 3500mg.

TOP RECOMMENDED POTASSIUM SUPPLEMENT:
==
MANUFACTURER: NOW FOODS
PRODUCT NAME: POTASSIUM CITRATE, 99 MG, 180 CAPSULES
WEBSITE: www.nowfoods.com
PRODUCT PAGE: www.nowfoods.com/supplements/ potassium-citrate-99-mg-capsules

Mineral supplements like Potassium Citrate can be DANGEROUS if taken in large amounts in one sitting because they are very highly soluble and enter the blood stream FAST and can mess with your blood electrolyte levels enough to CAUSE A HEART ATTACK. You can take a single Potassium supplement pill with any meal, but a single 100mg pill is just 2.8% RDA and the FDA prohibits the production of pills containing larger amounts because the Potassium mineral salts are so highly soluble and therefore dangerous. Start with the Low Sodium Original V-8 and bananas and try to get most of your Potassium from food sources ONLY.

26. SELENIUM: 70mcg/day – This is another trace mineral that the thyroid uses to build its critical hormones. Selenium also happens to be an antioxidant and although present in only trace amounts, it may serve to help relieve oxidative stress in the thyroid gland itself. Selenium deficiency while not as common as Iodine deficiency can also result in hypothyroidism which causes a marked decline in metabolism resulting in lethargy, fatigue, and ultimately obesity and inactivity which can result in sundry adverse consequences including high blood pressure, cardiovascular disease, and thyroid disease.[26]

BEST FOOD SOURCES – BRAZIL NUTS (2 nuts, 100%DV), MUSSELS (4oz, 145%), SHRIMP (4oz, 102%), SUNFLOWER SEEDS KERNELS (3oz, 96%DV), PORK (lean cut, top loin, 5oz, 85%), SARDINES (4oz, 84%), WHEAT GERM (2.5oz 80%), BEEF SIRLOIN (5oz, 80%), TURKEY (breast, w/o skin, w/o bone 6oz, 78%), COD (5oz, 75%), ATLANTIC MACKEREL (4oz, 72%) [32][43][60][62][65][95][96][117][132][141][149][151]

We only need Selenium in micrograms, but even that tiny amount makes a huge difference between being healthy and getting into serious trouble. Just TWO BRAZIL NUT KERNELS brings roughly the 100% RDA of this critical mineral. I consider them to be two tasty chewable Selenium supplements that make getting your Selenium from a natural source too easy to pass up.

TOP RECOMMENDED SELENIUM SUPPLEMENT
==

MANUFACTURER: NATURE'S WAY
PRODUCT NAME: SELENIUM, 200 MCG, 100 CAPSULES
WEBSITE: www.naturesway.com

Seeds, nuts and fish are the primary natural sources of Selenium. However, Beef Sirloin, Pork and Turkey Breast are also excellent sources although they do bring Saturated Fat and Cholesterol. If you are avoiding the seeds and nuts because they are high in calories, and meats because of the cholesterol then you might have to take a supplement. This one made by a quality company brings about three times more than the RDA and you could take one capsule every two or three days.

27. SODIUM: 2500mg/day – Sodium is involved in the same synapses as Potassium in what is called the "Sodium-Potassium Pump" which is what moves the electron from the brain signal across the synapse to the muscle which allows it to respond. Fortunately, almost no one ever suffers from Sodium deficiency and in excess it can and will lead to high blood pressure, but in deficiency it is even MORE LETHAL because acute deficiency results in rapid muscle twitching because the nerves can no longer control the muscle and if that happens to the heart it is called palpitations, and it can be fatal in mere moments.

BEST FOOD SOURCES – IODIZED or SEA SALT (½ tsp/daily)

If you have eliminated junk foods, packaged and processed foods and only buy "No Salt Added" canned goods then you can go back to adding ½ tsp of IODIZED or SEA Salt to your food daily and get the Sodium, Chlorine and Iodine your body needs. Many fish and other sea foods happen to be high in Sodium because they absorb the salt into their tissues and use it to equalize the osmotic pressure so they don't dehydrate from the salty ocean water. They also happen to be good sources of Iodine because it is prevalent in sea water as well. Bear this in mind if you eat a lot of fish and other sea foods.[27]

28. SULFUR: No RDA established – Although there is no RDA for sulfur, that is only because the FDA assumes that most people get enough of this critical mineral involved in several amino acids which means it is in every protein in every cell in the human body. Sulfur is involved in the amino acids that are used extensively in the construction of Collagen, a protein used in the connective structures in the joints. Sulfur deficiency is usually not the cause of painful joints, but rather Copper and Molybdenum deficiency which prevents the body from being able to utilize the sulfur which is common in most foods. However, it is still good to add foods high in basic sulfur compounds, this ensures that your body is getting plenty of this important mineral.[28]

BEST FOOD SOURCES – GARLIC, ONIONS, BROCCOLI, CABBAGE, BOK CHOY, CAULIFLOWER, BLACK PEPPER, MUSTARD, CHIVES, SHALLOTS, LEEKS, EGGS, FISH.

All of these foods are high in sulfur compounds and they stand out as the "stinky" foods because of their high basic sulfur content and they are excellent for your health. Just be sure to get some Molybdenum (from the legumes listed above) and Copper (many different foods) so your body can UTILIZE all of that sulfur. The only supplements available are not for sulfur itself, but for joint support such as Glucosamine Chondroitin, and both of these compounds contain sulfur, but in specific forms. The body can work with sulfur and build what it needs as long as you get good amounts of the supportive minerals as well.

29. ZINC: 15mg/day – Zinc is another big problem. We need almost as much as we do Iron, but it is not nearly as common as Iron in most foods and although many plant foods are loaded with it, some are also loaded with Phytic Acid and Phytates which have been shown to inhibit its absorption. If Iron is hard to get, you can bet that Zinc is nearly impossible to get from an unmanaged diet and the consequences are sundry and terrible: attention and motor disorders, nerve dysfunction (severe effect on the human brain and nervous system,) digestive problems, hormonal imbalance, impaired immune system, allergies and autoimmune disease, hypothyroidism, thinning hair, inability to absorb other nutrients, skin rashes and acne. [29]

BEST FOOD SOURCES – OYSTERS (canned, 1oz 170%DV), LAMB (5oz, 75%DV), DARK CHOCOLATE (100% pure 4oz, 72%), PUMPKIN SEEDS (4oz, 76%DV), WHEAT GERM (2.5oz, 60%), BEEF SIRLOIN (5oz, 55%DV), CASHEWS (3oz, 44%DV)

Other than oysters, no single superfood can provide you with 100% RDA of this critical nutrient involved in many enzymes within all of the cells in your body. Try to piece it together and make sure to get 100% RDA amount daily.[29][43][53][55][57][74][92][149]

TOP RECOMMENDED ZINC SUPPLEMENTS
==
MANUFACTURER: NOW FOODS
PRODUCT NAME: L-OPTIZINC 30 MG
WEBSITE: www.nowfoods.com
PRODUCT PAGE: www.nowfoods.com/supplements/ l-optizinc-30-mg-veg-capsules
==
MANUFACTURER: GARDEN OF LIFE
PRODUCT NAME: VITAMIN CODE RAW ZINC
WEBSITE: www.gardenoflife.com
PRODUCT PAGE: www.gardenoflife.com/content/product/ vitamin-code-raw-zinc/

Both of these quality products provide Zinc in a highly available form. The Now Foods product is a synthetic chelate shown to be very well absorbed in the digestive tract and the Garden of Life product is a natural source extract of the highest quality.

FINAL NOTE ON THE MINERALS

WATCHOUT – ALL MINERALS CAN BECOME TOXIC IN EXCESS WHICH IS EASY TO DO WITH SUPPLEMENTS: DO NOT EXCEED THE 100% RDA AMOUNT PER DAY OF ANY MINERAL FROM ANY SUPPLEMENT REGARDLESS OF ANY CLAIMS MADE ABOUT THE PRODUCT. DO NOT EXCEED AN AVERAGE INTAKE OF 100% RDA DAILY FOR ANY MINERAL FROM NATURAL FOOD SOURCES.

30. ALPHA-LINOLEIC ACID (the plant Omega-3: est. 500+ mg/day) – The Omega-3 Fatty Acids are essential nutrients but the body actually needs DHA and EPA (the next two in this list) not necessarily ALA. We can convert ALA into DHA and EPA, but we still don't know if the body can convert enough into the needed forms on a daily basis. There is no harm in getting plenty of ALA from natural foods or even supplements, but health professionals recommend getting DHA and EPA on a daily basis as well.[59]
BEST FOOD SOURCES – CHIA SEED (2457mg/Tbsp) FLAX SEED (1597mg/Tbsp) WALNUTS (1oz, 2600mg)[30][105][135]

Watch out for supplements labeled "ALA" because this acronym is used for other compounds like Alpha-Lipoic Acid (an Omega-6 Fatty Acid) which is definitely NOT the same thing.
31. DOCOSAHEXAENOIC ACID (DHA always found with EPA, the animal Omega-3's: est. 520mg/day) – Only in the past few decades have researchers come to realize that DHA and EPA are essential nutrients. Our body can convert alpha-Linoleic Acid (the plant Omega-3) into DHA and EPA, but that would still require an ample supply of ALA from plant foods, mainly seeds and nuts, which many people do not eat. Deficiency has been linked to: inflammation, higher risk for heart disease, high cholesterol, digestive disorders, allergies, arthritis, joint pain, muscle pain, depression, poor brain development, and cognitive decline. It looks like the FDA will set the RDA for a combination of both DHA and EPA at 520mg/day.[42]
BEST FOOD SOURCES – ATLANTIC MACKEREL (1oz, 750mg), SALMON (1oz, 575mg), SARDINES (1oz, 415mg), TUNA (1oz, 80mg) [42][59][60][61][62]

It is plain to see that the critical Omega-3's are a FISH thing. Many health professionals are recommending at least 1000mg/day and some recommend as much as 4000mg/day. Researchers have shown that the ratio of Omega-6 fatty acids (found in seeds, nuts and vegetable oils) to the Omega-3's is also important. The Omega-6's which are also beneficial to human health should be kept at no more than 5 times the amount of Omega-3's with a 2:1 ratio of O6FA's to O3FA's being ideal for decreasing inflammatory stress and maintaining healthy cholesterol levels and getting the most of the health benefits of both forms of nutritional fatty acids.

TOP RECOMMENDED OMEGA-3 SUPPLEMENT
==

MANUFACTURER: Any Reputable Brand
PRODUCT NAME: COD LIVER OIL (1Tsp/day)

Cod Liver Oil is one of the best natural supplements you could take bringing Vitamin A as Retinol, Vitamin D3, and 888mg of the Omega-3 Fatty Acids DHA and EPA. Fish Oil pills are acceptable but some health professionals have noted that Krill oil pills may be contaminated. Bear in mind that Olive oil is the only salad dressing you should use (Oil and Vinegar) and it is loaded with Omega-6's which will need to be balanced by Omega-3's as well. The Omega-3's are considered very safe nutrients; overdosing, even extreme amounts, has shown no adverse reactions or toxic effects.[59][71]

32. EICOSAPENTAENOIC ACID (EPA) – See DHA

33. ISOLEUCINE (19mg/kg) – This is the first of the nine essential amino acids that must be consumed in sufficient quantities on a daily basis because the body cannot manufacture them. This amino acid is involved in the formation of hemoglobin in the blood and muscle growth especially in children.[52]

34. HISTIDINE (14mg/kg) – Histidine is involved in detoxification of the body and is another critical component required to maintain healthy brain function.[52]

35. LEUCINE (42mg/kg) – Leucine, like all amino acids, is an integral part of many proteins used by all cells in the body but it is also used to moderate insulin levels and helps regulate blood sugar levels in the blood. [52]

36. LYSINE (38mg/kg) – Lysine is an "animal amino acid" and most plant proteins are deficient. Lysine is necessary for proper utilization of calcium in the body and promotes bone health.[52]

37. METHIONINE (+ Cysteine 19mg/kg total of both) – Methionine is a critical component of bone cartilage and helps in producing Creatine, a precursor to ADP – Adenosine Triphosphate – the main fuel used by muscle cells. The actual RDA is 19mg/kg of both Methionine and Cysteine which should both be acquired in proper amounts: about 13mg/kg of Methionine and 6mg/kg of Cysteine which alone is not considered essential (we can make it.) Methionine contains a sulfur atom and is generally deficient in plant proteins.[52]

38. PHENYLALANINE (+ Tyrosine 33mg/kg total of both) – Phenylalanine is used by the thyroid o produce its hormones and a dietary lack can result in similar deficiency syndromes to either Iodine or Selenium. Tyrosine which in not essential (we can make it) is involved in the construction of the Thyroid hormones and possibly other uses of Phenylalanine as well. No sources indicate the individual breakdown of the amounts of these two amino acids but they should be roughly 1-to-1.[52]

39. THREONINE (20mg/kg) – Threonine is a critical component of the central nervous system and it is important for heart and liver health and also plays a key role in the immune system.[52]

40. TRYPTOPHAN (5mg/kg) – Contrary to popular belief, Tryptophan does NOT cause drowsiness. If that were true then Chicken, which has a higher concentration of this important amino acid than Turkey, would make everyone sleepy too. Since it doesn't, Tryptophan cannot be the culprit. Ironically, Tryptophan is an important nutrient for the brain and adequate supplies are needed for the brain to build its neurotransmitter chemicals and maintain alertness and sharp memory. Chronic deficiency will lead to cognitive decline, memory loss, mood changes, sluggishness – the exact opposite of what most people believe. The reason folks get drowsy on Thanksgiving is because we generally eat far too much food especially the Turkey and massive overindulgence in protein and calories will make you drowsy.[52][166]

41. VALINE (24mg/kg) – Valine is well known to body builders and athletes and is necessary for muscle health and is involved in muscle growth, repair and endurance.[52]

COMPLETE PROTEIN (50g/day) – Virtually all foods have some protein in them, plant proteins are generally deficient in at least two of the nine essential amino acids: Methionine and Lysine.[52] The issue of "Complete Protein" and the nine essential amino acids is quite complicated and confusing. Aside from the fact that there are nine essential amino acids that cannot be manufactured in the human body, there are an additional six of them that are considered "conditionally essential." This means that in some circumstances (illness, injury, surgery, convalescence, pregnancy, heavy work, stress, etc) the body cannot make enough of them to keep up with the demand. Another problem with these amino acids is that the amounts required daily have been changed repeatedly especially in the past twenty years as more studies have been done yielding often radically different results. In addition, the World Health Organization and the U. S. Food and Drug Administration have published different recommended amounts of each one of them and the trouble becomes clear. Furthermore, these amounts are based on body weight alone which is still a "One size fits all" approach because a young man weighing 200lb but in excellent shape (i.e. a body builder) versus another who is not in good shape and elderly, must have distinct essential amino acid (and indeed all of the Big 43) requirements.

Finally, each food has a unique array of proteins; it is obvious that the proteins in Asparagus will be very different from those in a steak. But even within the animal kingdom, there can be significant differences not only in the proteins, but in the average amounts of the individual amino acids out of which they are built.

BEST FOOD SOURCES – To get all nine essential amino acids in sufficient quantities on a daily basis, animal meats are by far the best choice. All animal meats provide all nine essential amino acids and include: FISH, CHICKEN, TURKEY, LAMB, CLAMS, BEEF, SHRIMP, OYSTERS, CALAMARI, etc.

The amount of Complete Protein does vary dramatically from one meat product to the next especially in sea foods due to the water content. You cannot judge meats solely by the caloric content either (50g of Complete Protein will yield about 200 calories) because all meats also bring some amount of saturated fat which brings about 255 calories per ounce. The lower the amount of calories per ounce of the meat, the less fats and proteins, and the higher the water content. Try to stick to the leanest, lowest calorie meats that you can, this is the best way to avoid the saturated fats which tend to find their way to your thighs. Turkey breast is one of the best, or rather densest, sources of Complete Protein bringing 100% in 6 ounces while only bringing about 300 calories which is superb. As for cholesterol, there is no avoiding it; it is in virtually all animal cells, and some of the richest sources of Complete Protein are loaded with it because it is a critical component in the construction of cell membranes and it provides them with elasticity – the ability to change shape. This means it is highest in the skin and muscles including our own. The best way to deal with cholesterol is to reduce your total daily caloric intake of animal protein to the bare minimum requirement to get enough. Add high fiber foods as side dishes to these foods and add foods that help break down fats (Black pepper does this) and stimulate fat burning metabolism (Citrus fruits are good at this) and to drop all foods high in trash calories and chemical additives. The goal is to relieve the load on your liver so it can do its job: BUILDING and REGULATING the amounts and the forms of the cholesterols (LDL's and HDL's) it is putting into the blood stream.

42. ANTIOXIDANTS (No RDA established)

This is a huge category of phytochemicals. They are basically unique to plants and every major category of plant chemical from the terpenoids to the phenolics to the organic acids has members that are also powerful antioxidants. Most folks are aware that Vitamin C is a powerful antioxidant, but beta-Carotene commonly found in many plants is 25 TIMES more potent and Lycopene, which makes tomatoes and watermelon pulp red, is 40 TIMES more potent than Vitamin C. There has been a lot of hype over antioxidants but it is well deserved. Antioxidants "relieve oxidative stress" in virtually all cells in the body which in turn makes every organ system healthier by reducing cell death and increasing the vitality of every cell which makes the organs healthier and brings them up to OPTIMUM THRIVE-LEVEL health and performance.

"Relieve oxidative stress" in all cells means that antioxidants neutralize the metabolic waste by-products caused by burning carbohydrates and proteins. Proteins in particular are very dirty burning fuels that produce very toxic waste in the cells compared to the carbs which also produce toxic waste by-products. These can lead to a decline in the performance of the cell and even kill it when left unchecked. Unmanaged diets low in antioxidant-rich foods quite literally cause a build-up of these oxidants in all tissues and no magical detox product will help – only the antioxidants can transform your body from an oxidant-rich environment to a clean environment low in oxidants.

Numerous studies have shown that the antioxidants do serve as detoxification agents that improve the health and performance of literally every organ system in the body and reduce the risks of (help prevent) and even ameliorate the effects of just about every member of the BIG SEVEN modern epidemic plagues including but certainly not limited to: 1) Cardiovascular Disease, 2) High Blood Pressure, 3) High Cholesterol, 4) Alzheimer's disease, 5) Type II Diabetes, 6) Stroke, and 7) Cancer. And the vast majority of all cases of these terrible afflictions are the result of chronic poor diet starting with a shortage of antioxidant-rich foods.

The worst of all modern plagues is Cancer which CREATES and THRIVES in OXIDANT-RICH environments. It is therefore no coincidence that oxidant-rich environments ENCOURAGE its formation and proliferation while antioxidant-rich environments can dramatically reduce the risk of its formation and severely slow its proliferation. Do yourself a favor and load up on antioxidants.

I have included the ORAC (Oxygen Radical Absorption Capacity) Scores in parentheses with each food despite the fact that this is considered an obsolete form of measurement. This is because no two antioxidants are the same. Nevertheless, the same amount of each food is used in the test and it provides a convenient method of comparing the foods side-by-side even though there are more comprehensive methods of measuring them now (but they are not necessarily any more accurate.)

BEST FOOD SOURCES – Alfalfa Sprouts (1,510) **Apple** (4,275) **Apricot** (1,110) **Artichokes** (6,552) **Arugula** (1,904) **Asparagus** (2,252) **Avocado** (1,922) **Banana** (795) **Bean Sprouts** (962) **Beets** (1,776) **Bell Peppers** (935) **Blackeye Peas** (4343) **Black Raspberries** (19,220) **Blueberries** (4,669) **Broccoli** (3,083) **Brussels Sprouts** (1,330) **Cabbage** (boiled, 856) **Carrots** (raw, 697) **Cauliflower** (boiled, 739) **Celery** (552) **Cherries** (3,747) **100% Concord grape juice** (2,389) **Cranberries** (9,090) **Dark Chocolate** (unsweetened baking squares 49,944) **Elderberries** (14,697) **Figs** (3,383) **Gooseberries** (3,332) **Goji Berry** (3,290) **Grapefruit** (1,548) **Green beans** (799) **Green peas** (600) **Hazelnuts** (9,645) **Kale** (1,770) **Kiwi** (862) **Lemon** (1,346) **Lingonberry** (20,300) **Mulberries** (6,130) **Oranges** (2,103) **Peach** (1,922) **Pecans** (17,940) **Pineapple** (562) **Plum** (6,100) **Pomegranate** (4,479) **Prunes** (8,059) **Raisins** (3,406) **Red Cabbage** (Boiled, 3,145) **Red Grapes** (1,837) **Red Raspberries** (5,065) **Spinach** (1,513) **Strawberries** (4,302) **Tamarind** (3,500)

Tangerine (1,627) **Tea Leaves** (62,714 dried) **Tomatoes** (546) **Walnuts** (13,541)[34]

If it is raw antioxidant power you are looking for, the dried spices are at the top of the list and you should use them liberally in your cooking to take advantage of their incredibly high antioxidant potency and their powerful and often unique phytonutrients that deliver a wide range of proven health benefits.

THE SPICE RACK – THE ANTIOXIDANT POWERHOUSE –
Basil (61,063 dried, 4,805 fresh), **Black Pepper** (34,053), **Cayenne Pepper** (19,671 ground), **Chili Powder** (23,636), **Cilantro** (5,141 fresh), **Cinnamon** (131,420), **Cloves** (290,283), **Cumin** (50,372), **Curry Powder** (48,504), **Dill Weed** (4,392 fresh), **Garlic** (6,665 dried; 5,708 fresh), **Ginger** (39,041 ground,14,840 raw), **Lemon Balm** (5,997 fresh), **Marjoram** (92,310 dried), **Nutmeg** (69,640 ground), **Oregano** (175,295 dried; 13,970 fresh), **Paprika** (21,932), **Parsley** (73,670 dried), **Peppermint Leaves** (160,820 dried, 13,978 fresh), **Rosemary** (165,280 dried; 11,070 fresh), **Saffron** (whole, 20,580),**Sage** (119,929 dried; 32,004 fresh), **Savory** (9,465 fresh), **Star Anise** (11,300), **Tarragon** (15,542 fresh), **Thyme** (157,380 dried, 27,426 fresh), **Turmeric** (127,068 dried), **Vanilla Bean Spice** (122,400 dried), **Yellow Mustard Seed** (29,257)[34]

Most dried spices have immense ORAC scores because most of the water has been removed and water makes up about 85% of all plant matter except for seeds which are naturally desiccated and waiting to absorb water like a sponge in order to sprout; so they are already naturally dehydrated and concentrated and loaded with antioxidants. Dried fruits like raisins and prunes are also much higher in their ORAC scores for the same reason.[34]

After the spices most fruits and some nuts are the second best option and they too bring high antioxidant potency and also many other members of the Big 43 as well as their own unique phytonutrients that have also been proven to have sundry and significant health benefits.

Many antioxidants are available in supplement forms including beta-Carotene, Lycopene, Quercetin, etc, and numerous studies have shown that these powerful antioxidants become severely depleted during the extraction and processing; to be clear, most antioxidants become USELESS and INEFFECTIVE once they are extracted and processed into pills. This makes sense because most of them will react with the oxygen in the air which depletes them. Key exceptions to this rule are the oil soluble antioxidants which instead of being purified are allowed to remain in their oils like Vitamin E and natural extracts like Astaxanthin.

Many people overdose on synthetic Vitamin C tablets seeking the raw antioxidant power of the vitamin. But the body will remove it once it reaches certain concentrations in the blood so taking large amounts will not reap the expected rewards. For those who want high antioxidant intake in order to get in on the myriad health benefits of these compounds, rule #1 is: MORE IS NEVER BETTER WHEN IT COMES TO STRONG MEDICINE. Instead of overdosing on ONE antioxidant, the far better approach is to get as many DIFFERENT ones as you can. The plant kingdom (and by now you should realize that antioxidants are a PLANT thing) has thousands of them – there are over 1,100 tetraterpenoids alone which is just one class of phytonutrients that includes beta-Carotene and Lycopene. Since antioxidants are so easily depleted in processing, that means adding a variety of high antioxidant foods to your diet will be the most effective way to get in on their extraordinary and proven health benefits.

RECOMMENDED ASTAXANTHIN SUPPLEMENT
==

MANUFACTURER: SPRING VALLEY
PRODUCT NAME: ASTAXANTHIN 4MG, 30 GELCAPS
While this manufacturer may not be known for producing the highest quality supplements, their Astaxanthin comes from the natural extract of a species of Red Algae – it is a natural source extract which is excellent and recommended over synthetic forms. Astaxanthin is one of the most powerful antioxidants known to science and is about SIX THOUSAND TIMES STRONGER than Vitamin C. The 4mg in each pill delivers the same antioxidant power as FORTY EIGHT 500mg Vitamin C pills (the entire bottle of some products!) Astaxanthin won't disappoint; it is VERY strong and can actually deplete your immune system and make you vulnerable to infection, especially viruses like cold and flu. Bear this in mind if you shop around for other Astaxanthin products which are also available in 6mg, 10mg and even 12mg pills which would bring the antioxidant power of ONE HUNDRED AND FORTY FOUR 500mg Vitamin C pills in a single pill and they will severely deplete your immune system.

There is one antioxidant product that is even stronger than Astaxanthin, believe it or not, and it is called "Dragon's Blood" because it is very dark red. It is an extract from one of three different species of tropical bushes and all three extracts go by the same name and have similar antioxidant power, but if Astaxanthin 4mg is already so strong that it can threaten the immune system – I know from personal experience and only take ONE 4mg gelcap once or twice a week – then Dragon's Blood is obviously stronger and DANGEROUSLY high in antioxidants and should only be used at the recommendation of a medical doctor.

43. DIETARY FIBER (25g/day) –
Dietary Fiber is water-soluble and supports intestinal health and also bonds to cholesterol preventing its absorption in the digestive tract. A low Fiber diet can cause digestive difficulties and increase the risk of digestive tract disease including cancer especially colon cancer which is definitely on the rise likely due to low fiber intake.

BEST FOOD SOURCES – DARK CHOCOLATE (4oz, 76%DV,) BLACK BEANS (1 cup, 66%DV,) LENTILS (1 cup, 63%DV,) DRIED PLUMS (6.2oz, 49%,) CHICKPEAS (1 cup, 45%DV,) FAVA BEANS (1 cup, 38%DV,) AVOCADO (1 cup, 36%DV,) PISTACHIOS (3oz, 36%DV,) PECANS (3oz, 33%DV,) BLACKEYE PEAS (1 cup, 32%DV,) GREEN PEAS (1 cup, canned, 30%DV,) LIMA BEANS (1 cup, 30%DV,) SUNFLOWER SEED KERNELS (3oz, 30%DV,) WHEAT GERM (2.5oz, 30%DV,) PUMPKIN (1 cup, canned, 28%DV,) SWEET POTATO (1 cup, w/skin, 26%DV) [32][39][40][43][56][57][63][64][70][83][102][112][122][128][136][157] Because of its well known health benefits many people are now taking Fiber in any one of a whole store isle full of products. I always recommend getting your nutrients from natural whole foods first and fiber is no exception, and it is not difficult to get if you choose the right foods. But if you are going to supplement your Dietary Fiber intake, the best source is Psyllium seed and many products are available. Avoid products that only have the seed husks in them. While they are almost 100% Fiber, some reputable sources recommend products that contain the whole seeds in cracked form because the husks alone consist of so much Fiber that they are virtually impervious to our digestive tract and can cause digestive trouble when they are supposed to help prevent that. The cracked seeds provide more quantities of superior water-soluble Dietary Fiber than just the plain husks.[123][150]

TRACE MINERALS

Numerous studies are piling up linking Boron to superior health. Although it does not have an RDA yet, we already know that is fairly meaningless in the final assessment. All plants need Boron to support the meristems (the growing tips of new branches) and it is no surprise that we need it too. Foods richest in Boron are those plants that grow very fast (especially if we eat the growing stems) including: Asparagus, Black beans, Lima beans, Chick peas, Green peas, Green beans, Oats, Sunflowers, etc. And by the way, trace amounts of Boron can be added to the soils of these plants to help them grow faster, but even the slightest excess will kill them and excess Boron is likely not very good for humans either.

Another trace mineral that has been mentioned is Vanadium. It has also been mentioned as a possible plant requirement in exceedingly trace amounts, but the jury is still out regarding this one. One reliable source indicates that whole grains, fish and other sea foods as well as liver are the best sources. Since these are included in the Superfoods as well as the Natural Whole Foods Diet in the coming chapter, Vanadium in trace amounts should be adequately covered as well.

Another nutrient that is also being mentioned is Pangamic Acid, sometimes referred to as "Vitamin B15." Again, the research is ongoing, and it is present in significant amounts in Sunflower Seed Kernels: a true Superfood that you should incorporate into your regular eating regimen despite the high caloric content; they are worth it.

I have also seen a lot of fad products out there offering such things as Aluminum, Nickel or Germanium. Aluminum is a suspected cause of Alzheimer's disease and is very likely nothing more than a contaminant if it is present in foods at all. Even though it is abundant in the Earth's crust, it's oxides (aluminum ore) are some of the toughest molecules to break so it is unlikely that any plant would ever need it since it is not available in nature for their roots to absorb. Nickel is also abundant and a proven requirement for plants but in very trace amounts. When the amounts go up, the plants suffer and die. If we do need it, Nickel is another mineral likely needed in very small amounts because it is a known and DANGEROUS TOXIC METAL. And while I haven't looked into Germanium, it is again likely only needed in exceedingly small amounts if it is needed at all.

The bottom line on all of these, especially the weird elements, is to be CAUTIOUS. Just about every element in the periodic table can be found in the body, but they may simply be contaminants. Strontium, for example, is so chemically close to Calcium, that all biological systems mistake it for Calcium and incorporate it into the same roles where it does a fair job too. However, just because Strontium is found in the body, doesn't mean it is necessarily an essential nutrient, it is most likely there by accident, the mere coincidence that it is close enough to Calcium in chemical bonding behavior that all plants and animals mistake it for Calcium and use it like Calcium. As for the rest, if we do need them, it will be in tiny amounts that a varied natural whole foods based diet can easily provide. Taking supplements of these unusual elements and other fad compounds could easily lead to overdose and very likely bad TOXIC reactions and is therefore NOT RECOMMENDED.

MULTIVITAMINS

In a way, these are the worst possible dietary supplements ever invented. The main reason for this is that they cannot possibly provide you with all of the Big 43 that you need daily; and none of them do. Not counting the essential amino acids, sulfur, fiber or the antioxidants which are certainly necessary, but would ideally come from foods, the rest of the Big 43 essential nutrients in the preceding list total 12,124.911mg or 12.125 grams. Think about the physical size of a 500mg Vitamin C tablet. In order for a multivitamin to contain everything you need on a daily basis from Vitamin A to Zinc (the "A to Z" they always talk about) it would have to be physically the size of TWENTY FOUR of those pills; larger than a ping pong ball and I wouldn't want to have to swallow that thing. Furthermore, there is no way that a multivitamin could include all 3,500mg of Potassium. That would explode into your bloodstream altering your electrolyte balance and very likely CAUSE A HEART ATTACK.

Another terrible limitation to all store-bought multivitamins is that they contain only manufactured forms of the vitamins and minerals and a lot of these are being questioned by many health professionals concerning their "bioavailability" (if they can actually be fully absorbed by the digestive tract) and their safety (some synthetic nutrients have already been proven to be toxic, like all synthetic forms of Vitamin K, and others are suspected of being CARCINOGENS like Chromium picolinate.)

WATCHOUT – NEVER DEPEND ON OR BELIEVE THAT ANY MULTIVITAMIN WILL COVER ALL OF YOUR DAILY NUTRITIONAL REQUIREMENTS OF THE VITAMINS AND MINERALS: NONE OF THEM CAN SO NONE OF THEM DO.

But the real problem with these products is that many people buy them and diligently pop "one a day" and BELIEVE that they have covered ALL of their essential nutrients when that is quite literally IMPOSSIBLE. And to make matters worse, many of those vital nutrients are in terrible forms like the mineral oxides that have very low bioavailability (you do not actually absorb more than 10% of the amount listed on the label) or forms that are flat out TOXIC. Instead, go through the preceding list and try to find foods that can easily solve as many of the Big 43 as possible without having to take them as supplements. Iron is knocked out by canned clams. Just 1 oz. of canned boiled oysters brings 170%DV Zinc. Vegemite will bring more than sufficient amounts of Thiamine, Riboflavin, Niacin and Folate, four very important and difficult B Vitamins to get in at least 100% RDA amounts on a daily basis. And don't forget the Antioxidants and the Dietary Fiber. Together those two total well over an OUNCE of critical nutrients that you need. To be clear: since rounding up all eight of the B vitamins can be difficult, a natural extract source, quality B Vitamin Complex such as the Garden of Life product, is a far better supplement choice than a multivitamin. Most of the rest, especially Potassium, should come from well chosen foods.

CONCLUSION

From this list of the nutrients and the Superfoods, the best sources of the Big 43 essential nutrients, you can construct a widely varied diet that is high in nutritional value, fiber and antioxidants. I cannot stress enough how important a high fiber and antioxidant diet can be. Numerous studies including human clinical trials have already demonstrated incontrovertible proof that a diet high in antioxidants and low calorie foods will lower blood pressure, lower cholesterol, prevent or meliorate Type II Diabetes, cardiovascular disease and most forms of cancer and improve every organ system in your body. Diets high in fiber provide tremendous help to the intestinal tract and can reduce the risk of colon cancer as well as provide a much needed reduction in the amount of cholesterol absorbed in the digestive tract.

Four vitamins are NOT water soluble: Vitamin A as Retinol,

but beta-Carotene and other Carotenoids are water-soluble, Vitamin D3, Vitamin E (all forms.) and Vitamin K. Because these are FAT soluble, and not water soluble, they are much more difficult for the body to deal with than the water soluble vitamins (all of the B's and C.) You should not exceed the 100% RDA daily of Vitamin A (as Retinol) or the various forms of Vitamin E total. Vitamin A as beta-Carotene is however safe because it IS water soluble and an antioxidant in this form. Vitamin D3 is relatively safe in reasonable amounts but try to stay at 100% RDA daily.

Vitamin K as Phylloquinone (K1) from natural whole foods is relatively safe. We don't actually use it in the body. Instead the intestinal bacteria convert it into Menaquinone (K2) which is the form that we use throughout the body. There is a question about how much of the K1 that we eat is actually converted into K2 by those bacteria and it is likely never 100%. So there is already a limiting factor built-in to getting it from natural whole foods rather than supplements in the form of K2. 400% should be your daily maximum from natural whole foods but your weekly daily average should still be about 100%/day as long as you are getting at least 100% RDA of Vitamin E as well.

THE BOTTOM LINE

Some essential nutrients must come from natural foods: 1) The Nine Essential Amino Acids, 2) Vitamins A, B9, B12, and K, 3) The Antioxidants, 4) Phosphorus, 5) Sulfur, 6) Fiber, 7) Potassium, 8) Sodium, 10) Chlorine, 11) Iodine, 12) Copper, 13) Manganese, 14) Molybdenum, 15) Selenium.

You should make every effort to get as much as you can of the following from natural whole foods first and take supplements only to shore them up as needed: 1) Vitamins B1, B2, B3, B5, B6, B7, C, D, and E, 2) Zinc, 3) Iron, 4) The Omega-3 Fatty Acids DHA and EPA (and these O3FA's are the ONLY ones I recommend to be supplemented regardless of how much you get from foods.)

The following may be necessary in supplement form; try to stick to low serving sizes taken throughout the day (do not take the whole daily requirement amount of any mineral especially Calcium and Magnesium all at once): 1) Vitamin B7, 2) Calcium, 3) Choline, 4) Chromium, and 5) Magnesium.

Choline and Magnesium are both very tough to get in 100% RDA amounts on a daily basis from natural whole foods and I have yet to find natural source extracts of either. The mineral products of Magnesium are harsh and should be taken in low amounts at least three to four times daily to minimize their effects.

If you do not want to chase down a bowl of Vitamin B pills then get a high quality B Complex and try to avoid any such product that brings Vitamin B12 as Cyanocobalamin – that form tells you that the whole thing is synthetic and of cheap, inferior quality, and check to make sure that all of them, including Vitamin B7 – Biotin, are present and in at least 100% RDA amounts.

"Superfood" is another recent term that is often overused and "hyped." What constitutes a Superfood? Generally speaking it brings at least one essential nutrient in 100% RDA amount in a reasonable portion size. However, the term is being used for foods that bring a lot (not necessarily 100% RDA) of anything, including fiber (which is plant matter that can't be digested, but is admittedly still essential for optimum health,) antioxidants, etc. Foods high in fiber or antioxidants have enormous health benefits, but many of these foods should really be called "Functional Foods." This term means that the food brings more to the table than just calories. We need calories, they are the fuel for all cells in the human body, but there are too many foods in the modern diet that bring tons of calories and very little in the way of important nutrients that the body also desperately needs in order to function properly, stay healthy and achieve OPTIMUM THRIVE-LEVEL health.

Furthermore and of great significance is the fact that modern science has only just recently turned its attention toward the hundreds of compounds present in each natural plant and new discoveries concerning their often amazing health benefits are being made all the time. Many plants might not bring significant amounts of any of the "Big 43" essential nutrients, but instead bring their own array of powerful phytonutrients; chemicals that they manufacture for their own survival purposes, like the antioxidants, that modern studies and clinical trials are PROVING have significant positive impacts on our health and well-being. And there are thousands of edible plants out there many with dozens of unique compounds each, some that have already been shown in studies to have either positive effects on human health or real curative powers, but the work is still in its earliest stages. There are literally tens of thousands of identified naturally occurring compounds and perhaps even millions that have yet to be identified or properly tested to see what they can do for us. And since testing takes time and money, we may never know the full extent of what nature has to offer.

Although this is true, it is also true that the human body does recognize these compounds, the liver sees them and let's them pass through to the blood stream, and the cells see them and snatch them up and put them to use making us healthier. And at the same time, the liver also fails to recognize the many toxins that are being put into packaged and processed foods, and it treats them as they should be treated: as TOXINS, and stops them and sends them through the bile ducts to the colon for removal. Eating foods high in trash calories laced with these foreign (to nature) toxins, results in "irritating the liver" forcing it to stop what its doing to handle all of those junk calories, and to deal with those toxins and send a stream of highly concentrated poison to the colon;

hence the rise in colon cancer rates, and high cholesterol in modern society. The liver MAKES the cholesterol even if you never eat a single molecule of it in your entire life, and it sends it out into the blood in packets: LDL's – Low Density Lipoproteins, and HDL's – High Density Lipoproteins, for all cells in the body to grab and use to maintain and construct their cell membranes and grow. But the liver can't stay on top of that if it is constantly being interrupted by thousands of calories of poor quality foods being dumped into it throughout the course of the day.

This is where the power of the "Net Negative Calorie" foods comes to play even for those who are not concerned about their weight. Reducing foods high in trash calories with no significant nutritional value makes room for those foods that do bring good phytonutrients and significant amounts of the essential nutrients especially the seeds and nuts. These guys happen to be loaded with polyunsaturated fats which are concentrated calories, but they also bring concentrated nutrients as well.

The following list is certainly not comprehensive, but includes some of the richest sources of the Big 43 essential nutrients and can help you identify those foods that can bring them without having to rely on supplements which are often synthetic and of dubious reliability in terms of bioavailability and safety: especially the minerals, most of which are metals that can quickly turn toxic in excess. And this excessive intake that leads to POISONING is almost always associated with synthetic supplements and NOT natural whole foods.

Each natural plant food contains literally HUNDREDS of compounds that have been identified by science and unknown numbers of others that have yet to be identified. An excellent example of this is the recent detection of a NEWLY identified flavonoid called Fisetin, found in onions. Many such compounds were discovered long ago, but are only now being closely studied for their health benefits. Some compounds like Quercetin, a flavonoid discovered in Oak bark, are prolific in the plant kingdom; it is found in many edible foods ranging from Apples to Onions, and it is a powerful antioxidant and has very significant and scientifically proven health benefits.

Included in the Big 43 are two major classes of phytonutrient (things found in plants that promote health) that you should make every effort to get in high quantities from foods: Antioxidants and Fiber; specifically, Dietary Fiber. This refers to water soluble fiber, which has been shown to improve intestinal tract health and also reduces the absorption of cholesterol in the meal, both are highly desirable effects. Crude fiber, or water-insoluble fiber, can also be beneficial, but certain foods contain forms that are "antinutritional" or in other words they are detrimental to your health. No one eats grass all day due to the very high crude fiber content mainly in the form of cellulose. In fact, it's not good for cows either, but they do have huge quantities of bacteria in their stomachs that actually break down the cellulose in grass which is why they can eat it all day long. Another group of foods high in detrimental forms of crude fiber are the beans. Navy, Pinto, Kidney, etc, are all very high in bad forms of Crude Fiber, hence their reputation for causing "digestive difficulties," and although some do bring good amounts of beneficial nutrients, I recommend that folks should severely reduce or completely eliminate them from their regular dietary regimen. Beans are not evil, but there is a price to pay, and it is not worth it, when so many other foods bring ample amounts of the same nutrients anyway, without all of the bad crude fiber.

Not all beans are to be shunned. Lima beans and Black beans are both very nutritious and lower in crude fiber. A few other beans are also included in the following list of Functional Foods because they are, generally speaking, lower in crude fiber, bring significant nutrition or are Net Negative Calorie foods (less than 30 cal/oz.)

It is critical to get as much of the Omega-3 Fatty Acids, DHA and EPA as you can. This is one of the few supplements that I strongly recommend especially for those who don't eat fish very often, and these two powerful anti-inflammatory substances NEEDED by the human body are exclusively found in meaningful quantities in fish and other animal sea foods like shrimp.

Fresh fruits are some of nature's most powerful medicinal functional foods. Numerous studies aimed at individual fruits, have established their significant roles in human health and not just for their basic nutrition or even their antioxidant strength, but many have specific and unique phytonutrients in them that take active roles in our cellular biochemistry that promote health including Resveratrol found in grapes, Catechins found in apricots, bananas, and chocolate, and many others.

GLYCEMIC INDEX & CARB LOAD

Also included for many foods is their GI - Glycemic Index. This is a measure of how much sugar the food will quickly dump into your blood stream with pure Glucose scoring 100. Foods that score below 40 are to be considered the very best at keeping blood sugar levels in check. Most fruits score between 50 and 70 which is actually good considering the amounts of sugars they contain. Also included is CL – Carb Load. This is the percentage of the mass of the food that consists of sugars and starches. Obviously, the lower this number, the lower the food's impact on blood sugar levels. But there is no simple rule that can relate the GI to the CL because the GI is directly related to the exact forms of sugars and starches in the food. Potatoes, for example, are high in the kind of starch that once cooked is easily converted into sugars giving them very high GI's depending on the method of cooking of up to 80+ (worse than pure honey or watermelon) and no potato product scores lower than about 65. Rice and Corn, by the way, are no better and these three all get worse the longer they are cooked and the higher the heat of cooking, but even popcorn has a very high GI. Therefore, it is not the sugars and starches present in the food, but their forms and raw foods are always far better than cooked.[16]

COMPLETE PROTEIN, CHOLESTEROL, SATURATED FAT

Included with each food is a nutritional list that includes the physical amount of the food, its calories, and all members of the Big 43 that it brings in significant amounts (usually over 10% RDA amounts, however some are listed in percentages of the DV – Daily Value – amounts which have been determined by modern studies and differ from the RDA's like Biotin and Chromium.) Also included are the antioxidant ORAC Scores. Rather than list the essential amino acids, the amount of Complete Protein is listed instead, but every food's amino acid content is different and is covered in a later chapter in detail.

Since Cholesterol is a real issue I have listed the percentage of the "RDA" the food brings but I call it DL – Daily Limit instead because you don't want to reach 100% (which is 300mg.) The "RDA" for Saturated Fat is 20g/day and this is also treated as a DL – Daily Limit and the percentages are included for those foods (almost exclusively animal meats and some nuts) that have large amounts in them.

THE FUNCTIONAL FOODS

1. ALFALFA SPROUTS (and 2. Bean Sprouts) – 1 cup (1.2oz) = **8** cal, ORAC Score: 1510, CL: 0 (trace)

Talk about a Net Negative Calorie food! Although this list is in alphabetical order for easy reference, Alfalfa (and bean sprouts, usually Soybean or Mung Bean sprouts, by the way) have similar properties and are good place to start. Basically all of the nutrients in the seeds are present in the little spouted plants but in far superior forms. Admittedly they don't contain over 10% RDA of anything, but that doesn't take away from their broad spectrum of offerings and extremely low calories which is their greatest feature. Gone are the high calorie fats. Gone are the high quantities of Crude Fiber. Present are all of the other nutrients in an extremely low calorie food. Do NOT overindulge in Alfalfa though. It is great for horses and other grazing animals and gives them a big boost of energy which it does for us as well, but eating too much day after day will have BAD consequences. It is an excellent addition to tossed salad perhaps once a week. Bean sprouts have about the same calories (very few) and bring the same benefits (no fats, no Crude Fiber, and some of the nutritional content of the original beans, and added bonus: they don't mess with energy metabolism so you can eat them as often as you like and they are great for adding to soups, salads, stews and quick stir fried dishes.[75]

3. ALMONDS – (dry roasted) 3oz = **501** cal, 42% Vitamin B2, 185% Vitamin B7, 108% Vitamin E, 60% Magnesium, 51% Copper, 111% Manganese, 18% SATURATED FAT, ORAC

Score: 4454, CL: 5.6%[34]

Like all seeds and nuts, Almonds bring a lot of polyunsaturated fat – the good kind – and are therefore high in calories. However, they do bring plenty of nutrients making them a Functional Food. About 2oz will more than cover your DV for Vitamin B7 – Biotin, a rather hard one to get. Three ounces brings 108% RDA of Vitamin E and is a good reason to add these nuts to your weekly dietary regimen. They also bring 60% of the Recommended Daily Allowance of Magnesium, another member of the "Big 43" that is hard to get from foods. The antioxidant ORAC Score is excellent and likely due mainly to the high quantity of Vitamin E.[31]

4. APPLE – (raw) 1 cup (4.4oz) = **65** cal, 10% Vitamin C, 12% FIBER, QUERCITIN, RUTIN, URSOLIC ACID, ORAC Score: 2500 – 4200, GI: 39±3, CL: 10.5%[16][34]

Plain old apples are relatively low calorie and bring some much needed Dietary Fiber (the good kind.) Quercitin is a powerful antioxidant phenolic compound that has been well studied and has shown tremendous health benefits including: lowering the risk of atherosclerosis (plaque buildup in blood vessels,) lowering the risk of various forms of cancer, halting the growth of breast, colon, prostate, endometrial and lung cancers, lowers blood pressure, lowers several risk factors of heart disease, lowers cholesterol, and has shown success in the treatment of Diabetes, Cataracts, Hay fever and Asthma, Peptic ulcer, Schizophrenia and Mood disorders, Inflammation (prostatitis and interstitial cystitis,) Gout, Viruses (including H1N1, H3N2, H5N1, dengue, hepatitis B14 and C15,) Chronic Fatigue Syndrome, and circulatory problems. This very broad spectrum of health benefits is typical of many of these powerful antioxidants because virtually all cells in the human body recognize them and happily absorb them for the help they deliver. White apple products are far superior; when a processed apple product turns brown (like apple sauce) that means that the phenolics have been depleted and will no longer be as strong as they are in fresh white apple pulp.[77][159]

5. APRICOT – 1 cup (4.9oz) = **68** cal, 20% Vitamin C, 12% Vitamin A (as beta-Carotene,) 12% Copper, QUERCITIN, ANTHOCYANIDINS, CATECHINS, URSOLIC ACID, ORAC Score: 1110, GI: 34±3, Prunes: 29±4, CL: 9.1%[16][34]

Apricots are loaded with some powerful phytonutrients including: Quercetin, Anthocyanidins and Catechins which are of particular interest. These antioxidant flavonoids have been shown to: improve mood and psychological health, improve eye health, lower blood pressure, strengthen blood vessels, reduce fatigue, improve blood flow, reduce internal blood clotting, and strengthen the immune system. While the scientific community insists that there is little evidence to suggest that Ursolic Acid has significant health benefits, this Triterpenoid is suspected, and some preliminary research suggests, that it provides significant health benefits including: anti-inflammatory, liver protective, heart protective and anticancer properties. Various studies have demonstrated its ability to repair cognitive decline, to inhibit the proliferation of various cancer cell lines including JURKAT leukemia, to stave off muscle atrophy, to stimulate muscle growth, to stimulate neuronal regeneration after sciatic nerve damage, to induce cell death in deformed red blood cells, to enhance cellular immune function, to enhance pancreatic beta-cell function, to enhance endurance, to reduce fat cell accumulation (obesity caused by a high-fat diet) and to ameliorate Fatty Liver Disease. That's a lot of studies and a lot of exciting results. The added bonus is that you don't have to go out of your way or pay a fortune for it either: Apples, Apricots, Basil, Bilberries, Cranberries, Peppermint, Rosemary, Olives, Oregano and Thyme are excellent sources plus dried Apricots have even higher concentrations of this health promoting fruit's phytonutrients.[78][160]

6. ARTICHOKES – (boiled) 4oz. = **59** cal, 24% Vitamin B9, 20% Vitamin K, CAFFEOYLQUINIC ACID, ORAC: 4760,CL:1%[34]

Artichokes are certainly not at the top of many folk's list of foods they long for, however they are a respectable source of much needed Vitamin B9 – Folate and are a valuable source of a much needed and rather unique phytonutrient called Caffeoylquinic acid. This compound actively promotes liver detoxification and is one of the very best things you can feed to your liver. The good news for those who do not want to eat Artichokes, is that Artichoke Leaf Extract is the significant source of this compound and it is readily available in supplement form.[79]

7. ARUGULA – 1 cup (0.7oz) = 5 cal, 10% Vitamin A (as beta-Carotene), 28% Vitamin K, ISOTHIOCYANATES (sulfur compounds), CHLOROPHYLL, ORAC: 1904, CL: 2.1%[34]

If you get the chance to buy fresh Arugula, it is an excellent dark green leafy salad alternative. All dark green leafy vegetables are loaded with Chlorophyll which is the Number 1 Liver detoxification phytonutrient. Arugula also brings some Vitamin A as beta-Carotene and Vitamin K like most edible leaves. But its greatest health benefits come from the Isothiocyanates – sulfur-containing compounds that are potent antioxidants. These phytonutrients in Arugula have been shown to: reduce the risk of cancer, actively combat existing cancer, protect eye health and reduce the risk of Cataracts and Macular Degeneration, improve heart health and reduce the risk of heart disease, protect bone health, aid in weight loss, improve digestion, correct pH levels in the blood and tissues (Arugula is one of just a few Alkaline plant foods,) help prevent Type II Diabetes, improve blood cholesterol, and help reduce skin inflammation and infections. All of these benefits come from the Isothiocyanates and Carotenoids and Arugula is a close relative to Broccoli, Bok Choy, Cabbage and Kale, all of which have similar compounds and health benefits and are in this list as well.[80][161]

8. ASPARAGUS - (boiled) 1 cup (6.3oz) = **40** cal, 36% Vitamin A (as beta-Carotene) 20% Vitamin B1, 14% Vitamin B2, 10% Vitamin B3, 68% Vitamin B9, 24% Vitamin C, 14% Vitamin E, 114% Vitamin K, 14% Copper, 10% Iron, 14% Manganese, 10% Phosphorus, 12% Potassium, 16% Selenium, 10% Zinc, 14% FIBER, QUERCETIN, STEROIDAL SAPONINS, ORAC Score: 1644, CL: 1.3%[34]

Don't boil your Asparagus more than 3 minutes and don't store it more than two days either. Asparagus has a very high respiration rate (stays alive metabolizing compounds) up to five times higher than most other vegetables, and it also gets depleted of nutrients quickly when boiled. This means fresh is far better than canned. It does bring powerful and unique phytonutrients called Steroidal Saponins that are both fat-soluble and water-soluble and they get involved in key cellular biochemical processes and participate in strengthening the immune system and blocking certain processes that in turn kills cancer cells. Asparagus has been shown to lower cholesterol levels in the blood, especially the LDL's (the "bad" ones) and it is an anti-inflammatory which improves circulation and reduces risk of cardiovascular disease and has shown promise in fighting some forms of cancer. Other than Onions, no other food is higher in Quercetin than Asparagus (See Apples for details.)[82]

9. ATLANTIC MACKEREL – (baked) 4oz. = **230** cal, 40% Complete protein, 100% Vitamin D3, 52% Vitamin B3, 164% Vitamin B12, 13% Choline, 72% Selenium, 3000mg OMEGA-3 FATTY ACIDS DHA and EPA, **52**%DL CHOLESTEROL, 19%DL SATURATED FAT

Some species of the "oily" fish are very high in cholesterol. If you have high cholesterol, you might want to avoid them until you have that under control. However, these fish also bring tremendous health benefits starting with the "Big 43" essential nutrients. Mackerel is very high in Vitamin D3, the same one we make in our skin, which is hard to get from natural foods. It is also loaded with Vitamin B12, also in a natural form rather than a synthetic, and Selenium which is critical for Thyroid health. Finally, there is no food higher in the Omega-3 Fatty Acids DHA and EPA ounce for ounce than Atlantic Mackerel which easily earns this fish the title of "Superfood." Avoid canned Mackerel, there is some concern about heavy metal contamination in the canned products.[60]

10. AVOCADO – 1 cup (cubes, 5.3oz) = **240** cal, 42% Vitamin B5, 23% Vitamin B6, 30% Vitamin B9, 20% Vitamin C, 21% Vitamin E, 35% Vitamin K, 31% Copper, 36% FIBER, ORAC Score: 1922, CL: 0.8%[34]

Avocados are a rather unusual fruit. They are very high in a class of fats called Monounsaturated Fats. This gives them a lot more calories than most other fruits, but they do bring some unusual health benefits. Research has shown that these fats improve the absorption of Carotenoids like beta-Carotene. Foods very high in these outstanding antioxidants but low in fats like Carrots or the leafy greens like Kale and Spinach, or in Lycopene like Tomatoes, get a measurable boost in the delivery of their carotenoids when eaten along with Avocados. Furthermore, the studies revealed an amazing and unexpected additional effect: those carotenoids like beta-Carotene or beta-Cryptoxanthin which can be converted by the body into Vitamin A, get a boost in the conversion rate as well. Those special monounsaturated fats in Avocado have been shown to significantly lower cholesterol, provide anti-inflammatory and antioxidant support for the cardiovascular system (reduce risk of cardiovascular disease including Metabolic Syndrome linked to serious heart disease,) improve blood sugar regulation and reduce the risk of Type II Diabetes, and help with weight loss by improving satiety despite being loaded with calories. They make you feel full quickly and retain that feeling much longer than most other foods. The majority of the antioxidants in the Avocado are in the dark pulp closest to the peel, so the best practice is to slice them with the peel on, then peel each slice like a banana. This keeps more dark green pulp closest to the peel and you get more nutrients.[83]

11. BANANA – 1 large (4.8oz) = **121** cal, 20% Vitamin C, 25% Vitamin B6, 14% Potassium, 18% Manganese, 14% FIBER, CATECHINS, ORAC Score: 795, GI: 47 – 70 (depends on variety) CL: 17.6%[16][34]

Everybody knows that bananas bring Potassium, but not nearly enough to satisfy our huge daily requirement of this critical mineral. Nevertheless, two a day, in addition to Low Sodium Original V-8 brand vegetable juice can get the job done. Most people don't realize that bananas have a higher antioxidant potential than raw carrots and also bring a lot of Catechins (See Apricots for more details) Ever wonder why the Banana Split became the most popular and well known prepared ice cream dessert? The bananas and the chocolate fudge which are both loaded with Catechins. These compounds have been shown to improve mood and psychological health. How? The intestines starting at the end of the duodenum and all the way to the late colon are on the lookout to absorb all Catechins. They all go to the liver which takes full advantage of their enormous antioxidant power for its own well-being while converting them into even more potent forms called Epicatechins which it releases into the blood stream for all cells in the body to get. Even the brain cells reap the benefit of "Oxidative Stress Relief" (get a good cleaning away of built up oxidants) and thus your brain starts working better and therefore you, the person, start to feel better too. (See Dark Chocolate for more details.)[69]

12. BEEF LIVER – (raw) 3oz. = **113** cal. 33% Complete Protein, 285% Vitamin A (as Retinol) 135% Vitamin B2, 54% Vitamin B3, 60% Vitamin B5, 45% Vitamin B6, 60% Vitamin B9, 830% Vitamin B12, 50% (280mg) Choline, 24% Iron, **400%** Copper,

42% Selenium, 21% Zinc, 78%DV CHOLESTEROL, 6% SATURATED FAT.

Beef liver is a true Superfood and it comes highly recommended, but like most animal meats it is loaded with cholesterol so keep those portions in check. A 3oz. serving brings a lot of Vitamin A as Retinol and one of the highest amounts of Choline along with excellent amounts of many of the B Vitamins. It has a LOT of Copper in it which also means you should not exceed 3oz. per sitting twice a week.[48]

13. BEEF SIRLOIN (trimmed) – 5oz = **248** cal, 85% Complete Protein, 10% Vitamin B1, 15% Vitamin B2, 65% Vitamin B3, 10% Vitamin B5, 50% Vitamin B6, 35% Vitamin B12, 15% Iron, 10% Magnesium, 35% Phosphorus, 15% Potassium, 55% Zinc, 80% Selenium, 30% Choline, **15**%DL SATURATED FAT, **25**%DL CHOLESTEROL

While all of the strange and fancy foods are being touted by so many modern health professionals, I would still prefer a nice juicy sirloin steak or even a very lean Sirloin burger. And what do you know? It's got plenty of Zinc in it too. Not as much as Lamb and nothing comes close to Oysters, but most folks are much more familiar with beef and know how to cook it. Aside from the Zinc it also brings plenty of Vitamin B6 – a difficult one to get from natural whole foods and Beef will really help in this regard. Round that out with a big dose of Selenium and you can see that beef is not the evil it has been accused of being in recent years.[149]

14. BEETS – (canned) 1 cup (5.5oz) = **49** cal, 12% Vitamin B9, 11% Vitamin C, 16% Iron, 13% Sodium, 23% Manganese, 11% FIBER, BETALAINS, ORAC: 1776 (raw) CL: 5.5%[34]

Beets are a true Functional Food. They won't set records for providing the "Big 43" but they certainly help especially with Iron and Fiber, a unique combination of great benefit since many folks suffer from digestive problems with high Iron foods and especially high Iron supplements. They are a good very low calorie side dish that also brings Betaine (an amino acid) and a class of unique phytonutrients called Betalains making them worth adding at least one night a week to your regular dietary regimen. Betaine has been shown in studies to transform a common amino acid called Homocysteine in the blood into Cysteine and Methionine both of which are harmless and used by all cells to construct their proteins for growth and repair. However, unchecked concentrations of Homocysteine have been linked to dangerous cardiovascular diseases like atherosclerosis. Other studies have shown that the Betalains have neuroprotective and anticancer properties as well. Always look for any natural plant constituent that can provide protection to brain cells because I have known folks who suffered from Alzheimer's disease and it is a horrible way to go. Raw Beet Juice, available at some online dietary supplement retailers, is the best source of these Betalains.[84][162]

15. BELL PEPPER – (chopped, raw) 1 cup (3.25oz) = **29** cal, 16% Vitamin A, 16% Vitamin B6, 11% Vitamin B9, 157% Vitamin C, 10% Vitamin E, 10% Molybdenum, 7% FIBER, ORAC Score: 935 (Green var.) CL: 4.0%[34]

Bell peppers, a.k.a. Sweet Peppers, are a highly recommended "Net Negative Calorie" food and a great source of Vitamin C and a multitude of carotenoids which is why they come in almost every color of the rainbow. The brighter yellow, orange, red, and even dark purple ones are loaded with these powerful health promoting antioxidants. Carotenoids in general promote liver, eye and skin health and those many colors of Bell Peppers allude to the fact that they have a staggering array of them. I always emphasize that MORE is NEVER BETTER when it comes to strong medicine and also advise folks to take the "Shotgun approach" to nutritional health. This means instead of loading up on one good item, load up on as many different good items as you can. Bell peppers provide: Alpha-Carotene, Antheraxanthin, Beta-Carotene (See Carrots,) Capsanthin, Capsorubin, Cryptoflavin, Cryptoxanthin (See Egg,) Lutein and Zeaxanthin (See Kale,) Lycopene (See Tomato,) and Vicenin in varying amounts which depends on the variety. Now that's what I call a shotgun blast of these powerful tetraterpenoid antioxidants. Enjoy them fresh in tossed salads or added to soups, stews, etc.[85]

16. BLACK (TURTLE) BEANS – (canned) 1 cup (8.5oz) = **218** cal, 22% Vitamin B1, 17% Vitamin B2, 37% Vitamin B9, 11% Vitamin C, 23% Copper, 25% Iron, 21% Magnesium, 28% Manganese, 275% Molybdenum, 26% Phosphorus, 21% Potassium, 38% Sodium, 66% FIBER, ANTHOCYANIDINS ORAC Score: 6416, GI: 20 (dried, boiled) CL: 9.7%[16][34]

Black Beans are not just an exception to the rule about avoiding beans, they are a Superfood. They have a much lower ratio of Crude Fiber to Dietary Fiber than other beans and bring the 2nd highest amount of Dietary Fiber of any food in this list. They also bring significant amounts of many vitamins and minerals. Finally, Black beans have a very high amount of antioxidants in them called Anthocyanidins found in foods that are blue, purple, and red (See Blueberry for more details.) These compounds give the Black beans such an impressive ORAC Score (one of the highest of all beans.) Black beans have two very important properties aside from this: 1) Their unique starches are resistant to being broken down by our digestive processes and are only broken down by the probiotic bacteria of the large intestine which in turn provides energy to the cells of the large intestine and this lowers their "Glycemic Index" making them good foods for folks with blood sugar issues like hypoglycemia and Type II Diabetes. 2) They have some unique compounds that actually encourage cholesterol in the blood to return to the liver thus lowering blood cholesterol levels. While my source complains about their caloric content, they are in my "Net Negative Calorie" Foods list at about 25.5 cal/oz which is very good. Black beans are an excellent substitute for most other popular beans that have lower nutritional value and higher amounts of Crude fiber.[39]

17. BLACK PLUM – 1 cup (sliced, 5.8oz) = **76** cal, 11% Vitamin A (as beta-Carotene) 26% Vitamin C, 13% Vitamin K, 9% FIBER, ANTHOCYANIDINS, CHLOROGENIC ACID, ORAC Score: 7581[34]

Dark skinned plums owe their color to anthocyanidins, powerful flavonoid antioxidants (See Cranberries for more details.) But the health benefits of Plums and Dried Plums (a.k.a. Prunes) are just getting started. Chlorogenic acid is found in high concentrations in plums. It is a powerful phenolic antioxidant that neutralizes a very bad kind of oxidant found in the body called Superoxide Anion Radicals. Plums also protect cholesterol and fats from oxidative damage and since all cell membranes contain both cholesterol and fats this is a very useful property indeed. Plums also increase the absorption of Iron in the digestive tract. For those who are Iron deficient and want to avoid supplements that cause constipation, add foods high in Iron and precede them with a plum. The Crude Fiber in plums gets broken down by the intestinal bacteria into Butyric Acid, Propionic Acid and Acetic Acid all of which provide nourishment to the Colon cells. Propionic Acid has been shown to inhibit the enzyme the liver uses to make cholesterol and acetic acid is involved in many different processes (See Vinegar for more details.) Dried Plums which are basically concentrated plums, have a very good GI; so you can bet fresh ones score even lower (See Dried Plums for more details.)[157]

18. BLACKEYE PEAS – (canned) 1 cup (8.5oz) – **185** cal, 12% Vitamin B1, 10% Vitamin B2, 31% Vitamin B9, 11% Vitamin C, 14% Copper, 17% Magnesium, 34% Manganese, 17% Phosphorus, 12% Potassium, 30% Sodium, 11% Zinc, 13% Iron, 32% FIBER, ORAC Score: 4343 (raw) GI:38 (cooked w/salt) 52 (w/o salt) CL: 10.3% [16][34]

Raw Blackeye peas have over SIX TIMES the antioxidant power of raw carrots which is impressive. They are a source of Magnesium, a mineral difficult to get in most foods and also an excellent source of Dietary Fiber. Cooking your own, rather than canned Blackeye peas, will yield lower Sodium content and superior nutrition across the board. However, trials seemed to show a significant reduction in Glycemic Index when cooked with salt. Like most high fiber foods, Blackeye peas are very filling which lowers the total amount of food consumed during the meal and also reduces the urges to snack thereafter.[40]

19. BLUEBERRIES – 1 cup (5.2oz) = **84** cal, 32% Vitamin K, 22% Manganese, 19% Vitamin C, 13% FIBER, 9% Copper, ANTHOCYANIDINS, PTEROSTILBENE, ORAC Score: 4669, GI: 53±7, CL: 9.9%[16][34]

Often maligned and included in the lists of the top foods not to eat because of their thin skins and high pesticide contamination, blueberries are simply too good to pass up. Blueberries have a high amount of antioxidants primarily due to the Anthocyanidins which are what give them their striking blue color. This class of antioxidants has been shown to: improve liver, eye and skin health, lower blood pressure, lower cholesterol, and lower the risk of cardiovascular disease. Blueberries also contain two powerful Stilbenoids called Resveratrol (See Grapes for more details) and Pterostilbene, Studies have shown that Pterostilbene is a powerful anti-inflammatory, antioxidant, prevents and combats Diabetes, protects the heart, protects nerves and brain cells from damage, protects the cells in the body from damage to their DNA caused by chemical toxins, reduces the risk of cancer, and halts the growth of many forms of cancer. Because of these extraordinary powers, even blueberries tainted with pesticides are worth the risk because their constituents like Pterostilbene have been proven to protect your cells from chemical toxins. The FDA tested thousands of Blueberry products carrying the "Organic" label and only found a few tainted with pesticides so that is definitely the way to go and you should still wash them thoroughly.[41]

20. BOK CHOY – 1 cup (cooked, 6oz) = **20** cal, CL: **0.8**%, 40% Vitamin A, 16% Vitamin B6, 17% Vitamin B9, 59% Vitamin C, 10% Iron, 16% Calcium, 10% Manganese, 13% Potassium, 6% FIBER

Bok Choy is a member of the Brassica family of vegetables (See Cabbage for more details) and is rich in Glucosinolates: sulfur-containing compounds. In fact, over 70 antioxidants have been identified in Bok Choy and its many health benefits include: lowers blood pressure, lowers cholesterol, reduces risk of cardiovascular disease, and reduces the risk of cancer. Whether sautéed briefly in Olive Oil or boiled briefly (added late) in stews, Bok Choy is an excellent Net Negative Calorie vegetable with almost no sugars or starches in it making it a suitable vegetable for those with Diabetes that brings a lot of powerful phytonutrients, antioxidants, and good health benefits.[86]

21. BRAZIL NUTS –1oz = **183** cal, 24% Copper, 26% Magnesium, 17% Manganese, 20% Phosphorus, 767% Selenium, **21**% SATURATED FAT, ORAC:1419, CL: 2.5%[34]

Brazil nuts have the highest amount of Selenium of all foods. Just two kernels contain about 100% RDA of this critical mineral. And that's a good thing because even though the Omega-6 Fatty Acids are good for human health, just one ounce of these wonderful nuts brings over 27,000mg. I have them on hand and when I realize that I haven't eaten any Selenium-rich foods during the day, I have two of them. They are a convenient way to cover your Selenium requirement for the day. And don't worry about whether their soil has been depleted from cultivation. Brazil nut trees are one of the largest species of tree on Earth reaching heights of up to 170 feet and they take up to 40 years to mature and bear these wonderful nuts. They form the top canopy of the Brazilian rain forests and most of the world's supply comes from those trees. Like all nuts, they bring a lot of calories but are low in sugars and starches and won't severely affect blood sugar levels.[59][65][71]

22. BROCCOLI – (boiled) 1 cup (5.5 oz) = **55** cal, 13% Vitamin A (as beta-Carotene) 15% Vitamin B2, 19% Vitamin B5, 18% Vitamin B6, 42% Vitamin B9, 135% Vitamin C, 15% Vitamin E, 245% Vitamin K, 15% Choline, 53% Chromium, 13% Manganese, 15% Phosphorus, 10% Potassium, 18% FIBER, ORAC Score: 2160, CL: 1.4%[34]

Broccoli is a mainstay for a healthy diet. I have always loved it even as a kid and I am well aware that I am in the minority. But without Broccoli you will be very hard pressed to get sufficient amounts of Chromium in your weekly dietary regimen. Garlic can help, but no one – not even me, and I use it heavily – eats enough to get their fill of this critical mineral. Broccoli is also loaded with Sulfur-containing compounds which are used to build Collagen, a protein used not only in hair and nails, but also connective tissues including tendons and ligaments in the joints. Finally, Broccoli has an excellent amount of antioxidant power, a surprisingly high amount of Vitamin C and makes a good contribution to your daily intake of Dietary fiber.[49]

23. BRUSSELS SPROUTS – (boiled) 1 cup (5.5oz) = **56** cal, 14% Vitamin B1, 16% Vitamin B6, 23% Vitamin B9, 129% Vitamin C, 243% Vitamin K, 15% Choline, 14% Copper, 10% Iron, 15% Manganese, 12% Phosphorus, 11% Potassium, 320mg OMEGA-3 FATTY ACID ALA, GLUCOSINOLATES, 16% FIBER, ORAC Score: 1330, CL: 1.7%[34]

This is another notoriously avoided vegetable that brings a wide assortment of nutrition and good health benefits aside from the usual: low calories and high antioxidant power. Brussels sprouts have the highest amounts of Glucosinolates: sulfur-containing compounds (See Cabbage for more details.) more than any other commonly available cruciferous vegetable. In fact, they have a rare compound called 3H-1,2-dithiole-3-thione that is currently under investigation. Brussels sprouts have been shown to lower cholesterol, support liver function, support body detoxification, protect cellular DNA from damage, reduce the risk of cancer, optimize the body's native antioxidant system, reduce the risk of heart disease, reduce the risk of cardiovascular disease, support the digestive tract and improve colon health, and have significant anti-inflammatory power due to the unusually high amounts of anti-inflammatory compounds in them including some of those sulfur compounds, Vitamin K, and Alpha-Linoleic Acid (the plant Omega-3 Fatty Acid.) Brussels sprouts are far more potent medicine if steamed rather than boiled, but you can still get in on their very high quantities and greater numbers of different and unique sulfur compounds even from the canned product.[87]

24. BUCKWHEAT – (cooked) 1 cup (5.8oz) = **155** cal, 30% Manganese, 28% Copper, 20% Magnesium, 17% Phosphorus, 16% FIBER, RUTIN, LIGNANS, CL: 17.2%

Although most folks think this is a grain, it is actually the seeds of the plant which is not a grass like the true grains. Nevertheless, it is a very healthy alternative for most grains because it has fewer calories and is a popular breakfast "cereal." The compounds found in this healthy grain substitute have been shown in studies to lower cholesterol, strongly improve blood sugar regulation and reduce the risk of Type II diabetes. In fact, it is so effective at this that researchers in Canada are trying to develop strains with higher concentrations of the antioxidant flavonoid called Rutin which is largely responsible for this effect. Plant Lignans are found in many plant foods but have the highest concentration in whole grains and Buckwheat. They are converted by the intestinal bacteria into "mammalian lignans" which studies have shown protect the body against hormone-dependent forms of cancer including breast cancer and also protect against heart disease.[88]

25. BUTTERNUT SQUASH – (boiled) 1 cup (7.2oz) = **82**cal, 457% Vitamin A (as beta-Carotene, one of the best sources) 10% Vitamin B1, 10% Vitamin B3, 13% Vitamin B6, 10% Vitamin B9, 52% Vitamin C, 13% Vitamin E, 15% Magnesium, 18% Manganese, 17% Potassium, 16% FIBER, ORAC Score: 396, CL: 9.7%[34]

This is another excellent member of the Curcubits (cucumbers and their relatives) and it brings plenty of Vitamin A as beta-Carotene (despite the deceptively low ORAC Score) and compares well to other commonly available foods even carrots. Beta-Carotene is a potent anti-inflammatory and can reduce symptoms and help prevent many common afflictions triggered by inflammatory activity in the body including cardiovascular disease and arthritis. Both Vitamin A and C are known to help promote a strong and healthy immune system. The carotenoid antioxidants in Butternut squash have been shown to reduce the risk of cancer and Butternut squash has a unique protein that studies have shown to halt the growth of certain forms of melanoma skin cancer. You can't go wrong incorporating this low calorie Superfood into your weekly diet.[89]

26. BUTTON MUSHROOMS – (raw) 1 cup (3oz) = **23** cal, 25% Vitamin B2, 17% Vitamin B3, 13% Vitamin B5, 22% Copper, 10% Phosphorus, 11% Potassium, 32% Selenium, 6370mg BETA-GLUCANS, ORAC: 691 – 968, CL: 3.5%[34][155]

Plain white Button mushrooms and Portabella mushrooms are varieties of the same species, Agaricus bisporus, and are readily available in most well stocked grocery stores, both fresh and canned. Although this species has far lower levels of a special group of compounds called Beta-Glucans than most of the other gourmet edible mushrooms like Maitake, Shiitake, Reishi, etc, they do have them and they have been shown in numerous scientific studies to have extraordinary health benefits including significant immunostimulant power, and they also assist chemotherapy in combating certain forms of cancer. All edible mushrooms are best eaten raw or briefly sautéed in oil to prevent the loss of their antioxidants and the disintegration of these valuable Beta-Glucans which are actually unusual forms of complex sugar molecules. Cooking these mushrooms until they turn rubbery destroys most of both groups of powerful health promoting phytonutrients. Don't underestimate the verified and powerful health benefits of the Beta-Glucans, all edible mushrooms are to be considered Top Recommended Superfoods because of their immunostimulant power and their ability to help fight many different cancer cell lines. Supplements abound but most are "Fractions" or partial extracts of dubious quality and effectiveness. If you can find 100% pure dried powders or "unfractionated" extracts, those are the way to go, but be warned: all of the gourmet mushroom prices have skyrocketed since science has begun to verify their extraordinary and potent health benefits.[90]

27. CABBAGE – (boiled) 1 cup (5.3oz) = **35** cal, 94% Vitamin C, 204% Vitamin K, 12% FIBER, GLUCOSINOLATES, ORAC Score: 856 (boiled) CL: 3.6%[34]

Cabbage is the main representative of a large group of vegetables called the Brassica family (a.k.a. the "cruciferous" vegetables) and they all have high concentrations of Sulfur-containing compounds called Glucosinolates with a wide range of impressive health benefits. Cabbage itself brings more Vitamin C per ounce, per calorie, and per dollar cost than any citrus fruit. It has a higher antioxidant potential than raw carrots and is a very low calorie food. To top it off, Cabbage is also very high in Vitamin K and two of those sulfur compounds called Sinigrin and Glucobrassicin. The body converts both of these into other compounds that have been shown to have very significant power to prevent and combat bladder, colon and prostate cancer. Add it all up and Cabbage is a true Superfood. Aside from being the second least expensive fresh vegetable (after potatoes) only about 30% of its nutritional content is lost from being boiled until soft while most other vegetables lose much more making Cabbage one of the best foods on Earth.[37]

28. CANTALOUPE – 1 cup (cubes, 5.6oz) = **54** cal, 30% Vitamin A (as beta-Carotene) 58% Vitamin C, 5% FIBER, ORAC Score: 319, CL: 7.3%[34]

Don't be fooled by the deceptively low ORAC Score, Cantaloupes do have a lot of carotenoids in them, hence the quantity of Vitamin A. The main health benefit of Cantaloupes was demonstrated in a study showing very strong reduction of inflammatory markers in the blood along with a reduced risk of Metabolic Syndrome, a malady that can result in serious heart disease. Cantaloupes are not generally appreciated especially by the young who consider it an "Old Fogey" fruit (I didn't like them much when I was young either) but they are a low calorie fruit that can certainly be added into a home made fruit salad bowl in order to get in on their proven health benefits.[91]

29. CARROTS – (raw) 1 cup (4.5oz) = **52** cal, 428% Vitamin A, 20% Vitamin B7, 14% FIBER, ORAC: 697, CL: 6.8%[34]

Although carrots bring vast amounts of Vitamin A, it is in the form of Beta-Carotene which is NOT actually Vitamin A. It is a very strong antioxidant, about 25 times more potent than Vitamin C. Beta-Carotene, and several other related tetraterpenoids, can be converted by the liver into Vitamin A on demand and the added bonus is that you cannot overdose on them, while true Vitamin A as Retinol is definitely dangerous if taken in excess. Carotenoids as a group have been shown in numerous studies to reduce the risk of Type II Diabetes, reduce the risk of cardiovascular disease, improve liver, skin and eye health, and reduce the risk of most forms of cancer. The liver, skin and eyes greedily absorb beta-Carotene from the blood when it is available and this greatly improves these organ systems health. Raw carrots are a superb low calorie snack alternative to greasy, starchy potato chips, and provide a lot of help for more than your eyes.[38]

30. CASHEWS – 3 oz. = **464** cal, 206% Copper, 59% Magnesium, 61% Manganese, 71% Phosphorus, 44% Zinc, 8% FIBER, **32.6**% SATURATED FAT, ORAC Score: 1948, CL: 5.9[34]

Even though Cashews are not as noteworthy as many other nuts for their nutritional content, they do bring a lot of Zinc, one of the more difficult minerals to get on a regular basis. Like all nuts they do bring a lot of calories, but most are polyunsaturated fats which are far healthier and loaded with Omega-6 Fatty Acids which are anti-inflammatory and promote superior health. Cashews have been shown to help reduce blood triglyceride levels (a component of the blood that contributes to high cholesterol) and many health professionals are starting to advocate the benefits of Cashews for cardiovascular health.[71][92]

31. CAULIFLOWER – (cooked) 1 cup (4.4oz) = **29** cal, 13% Vitamin B5, 12% Vitamin B6, 14% Vitamin B9, 73% Vitamin C, 19% Vitamin K, 11% Choline, 210mg OMEGA-3 FATTY ACID ALA, 10% FIBER, GLUCOSINOLATES, ORAC Score: 739, CL: 1.9%[34]

Cauliflower is another "cruciferous" vegetable meaning it is in the Brassica family like Broccoli and Cabbage and is high in sulfur-containing compounds called Glucosinolates (See Cabbage for more details.) It is an unusual vegetable in that it contains high amounts of Choline, a very difficult nutrient to get from natural whole foods because we need a lot of it and it usually comes from foods high in saturated fat and cholesterol. It is also high in Alpha-

Linoleic Acid, the plant Omega-3 usually only found in significant amounts in seeds and nuts. These two essential nutrients already place Cauliflower in the important Functional Food category but add to that its incredibly low caloric content, high Fiber content, high antioxidant content, and those sulfur compounds and it is definitely an important part of a healthy diet. Regular consumption of Cauliflower has been shown to reduce the risk of cancer, cardiovascular disease, support the digestive tract, improve the immune system and provide anti-inflammatory and detoxification properties. Try not to overcook it by boiling which depletes its rich nutritional value quickly. Instead try steaming it for ten minutes. Another good way to prepare it is a short sauté on low heat in healthy oil such as Olive oil, Sesame seed oil or Coconut oil.[93]

32. CELERY (raw) – 1 cup (3.5oz). = **17** cal, 12% Vitamin A (as beta-Carotene) 40% Vitamin K, APIOLE, APIGENIN, 6% FIBER, ORAC Score: 552, CL: 1.8%[34]

Celery is the ultimate healthy alternative snack food. It brings almost no calories to speak of, and is loaded with two powerful phytonutrients called Apiole and Apigenin which in the past were front line prescription treatments for women's hormonal issues that have since been replaced by modern more expensive synthetic drugs. Studies have shown that Celery increases endurance during work, exercise and athletics and that is just the beginning of its health benefits. It is also a diuretic (prevents water retention) and increases fat metabolism which can help you lose excess weight or stay trim.[81]

33. CHICKEN – (breast, boneless, skinless, baked) 4oz. = **124** cal, 52% Complete Protein, 64% Vitamin B3, 24% Vitamin B6, 16% Choline, 20% Phosphorus, 28% Selenium, **20**% CHOLESTEROL, 2% SATURATED FAT

Baked chicken breast with the skin and excess fat removed is a very healthy and widely available food that brings a lot of Vitamin B3 – Niacin, and Vitamin B6 – Pyridoxine which are both rather difficult to get in a Natural Whole Food diet. This is the leanest way to include chicken in your diet bringing only 124 calories in 4 ounces barely missing the Net Negative Calorie foods list although admittedly, most preparations will probably have a few more calories than that, but it is still an excellent meat that brings a lot of Complete Protein (the Nine Essential Amino Acids.)[94]

34. CHICKEN LIVER – (organic, raw) 3oz, = **97**cal, 27% Complete Protein, 186% Vitamin A (as Retinol) 87% Vitamin B2, 42% Vitamin B3, 51% Vitamin B5, 36% Vitamin B6, 123% Vitamin B9, 231% Vitamin B12, 30% Choline, 21% Copper, 42% Iron, 24% Phosphorus, 66% Selenium, 15% Zinc, and **96%**DL CHOLESTEROL, 6%DL SATURATED FAT

There is no denying the nutritional value of liver. Just 3 ounces of Chicken liver will load you up on the B vitamins especially B2, B5, B6 and B9 which are notoriously hard to get from natural whole foods. However, those 3 ounces will bring ALL of your Cholesterol for the day and those with high cholesterol might want to steer clear until they have that under control. The obvious side dish to accompany Chicken liver is Black Beans or Lentils both of which bring a lot of Dietary Fiber, which helps to block the absorption of Cholesterol in the intestines, and far more antioxidants than most other foods which also reduces the bad effects of Cholesterol in the blood stream.[95]

35. CHICKPEAS (Garbanzos) – (boiled) 1 cup (5.8oz) = **269** cal, 71% Vitamin B9, 29% Copper, 26% Iron, 20% Magnesium, 84% Manganese, 270% Molybdenum, 17% Zinc, 45% FIBER, ORAC Score: 847, GI: 10 (fresh cooked) 38 (canned)[16][34]

A true SECONDARY FOOD by definition that must be cooked in order to become edible (raw chickpeas are harder than human teeth; you would literally chip, crack and split your teeth trying to eat them raw!) While a bit higher in calories than the "Net Negative Calorie" foods, Chickpeas nevertheless are very high in nutritional value bringing a lot of Dietary Fiber, Folate (Vitamin B9) and a good three days worth of Molybdenum in just one cup. Aside from its nutritional value which is quite impressive, the health benefits of eating Chickpeas are remarkable. The high Fiber content helps people feel full faster and for a longer time after consumption which leads to less food consumed in the meal and less tendency to snack between meals and they are a great addition to the Natural Whole Foods Diet as a way to cut caloric intake despite bringing a bunch themselves. It's Insoluble or Crude Fiber content is rather high, yet the form can be broken down by the probiotic bacteria in our digestive tract forming Short Chain Fatty Acids which provide much needed fuel to the Colon cells and there is evidence that they can also reduce the risk of Colon cancer. One study showed that just 1/3 of a cup daily over a few weeks led to marked improvement of insulin secretion and blood sugar levels. Regular consumption of Chickpeas has also been shown to lower total Cholesterol levels in the blood as well as both LDL's (the "bad" ones) and Triglycerides. The added bonus of Chickpeas is that you can make your own Hummus even from the canned ones although finding "No Salt" added products might be a bit of a challenge. Just mash them up in a mixing bowl along with a heaping teaspoon of minced garlic and some black pepper and a tablespoon of Olive Oil (or Sesame Seed Oil or even Extra Virgin Coconut Oil) and you have a superb healthy dip for your healthy snack foods like Celery and Carrots.[63]

36. CLAMS – (canned) 3.25oz. (1/2 can) = **134** cal, 45% Complete Protein, 13% Choline, 130% Iron, 1498% Vitamin B12, 360mg OMEGA-3 FATTY ACIDS DHA/EPA, **20%** CHOLESTEROL, 1% SATURATED FAT

Clams are a true Superfood. The good news is that even canned clams are mostly wild-caught and therefore loaded with nutrients.

No other food on Earth has such a high concentration of Vitamin B12 and since canned clams are inexpensive, there is no reason for anyone to settle for taking store bought synthetic Vitamin B12 which is NOT the same form found in nature. Bear in mind they do bring Cholesterol like all animal meats, so don't pile on other high cholesterol foods on the same day. Instead stick to high Fiber foods that can help reduce Cholesterol absorption.[54]

37. COCONUT (38. and Coconut Oil) – 1oz (oil) = **245** cal, **122**% SATURATED FAT, MCT's, ORAC Score: 1090[34]

The health benefits of Coconut Oil are impressive, but the very best results will come from Extra Virgin or Cold Expeller pressed Coconut Oil rather than Refined Coconut Oil or worse "Neutral" Coconut Oil that has been refined to the point of being flavorless. The refined oils have lost most of their powerful phytonutrient content. Coconut Oil does contain a lot of calories and it does bring a boat load of Saturated Fat, but it is still far better than animal fat. There is a lot of scientific interest in Coconuts and their Oil which contains Medium Chain Triglycerides (MCT's) including Lauric, Capric and Caprylic Acids which are some of the rarest and yet strongest nutritional fatty acids in nature that have been shown in studies to possess: antimicrobial, antifungal (kills Candida, a common infection,) anti-inflammatory, and immunostimulant properties. They also: prevent bone loss and osteoporosis, protect brain cells, are a sleep aid, improve brain function and mood, help prevent and fight certain forms of cancer, promote fat burning metabolism, provide thyroid and adrenal gland support which helps balance bodily hormonal levels, support digestion by killing bad bacteria while nourishing the probiotic good bacteria in our intestines, help stabilize blood sugar levels and prevent Type II Diabetes, lower Cholesterol levels, lower LDL's and increase HDL's in the blood, can eliminate constipation, and help prevent heart disease. Although most studies are in the early stages, there is no denying the tremendous power of these rare phytonutrients in Coconut Oil. In addition, it is very stable at high temperature making it ideal for cooking and you can use it instead of other oils in most applications especially if you find Olive Oil too bitter. In fact, the health benefits of Coconut Oil are similar to those of Olive Oil but it is more powerful and a wise addition to your kitchen.[104]

39. COD – (raw fillet) 5oz. = **115** cal, 50% Complete Protein, 30% Vitamin B6, 110% Iodine, 25% Phosphorus, 75% Selenium, 17% Choline, 310mg OMEGA-3 FATTY ACIDS DHA and EPA, **15**% CHOLESTEROL, 1% SATURATED FAT.

Cod is a great food for three very good reasons: 1) It is extremely low calorie for a meat bringing Complete Protein, 2) It brings the all-important Omega-3 Fatty Acids DHA and EPA and 3) It is one of the richest food sources of Iodine other than certain oceanic algae like Kelp. Personally, I prefer a baked Cod fillet to seaweed. Other than seeds and nuts you will be hard pressed to find a good source of Selenium and those nuts have far more calories than Cod. To top things off, Cod brings about 66% of the RDA amount of the Omega-3 Fatty Acids DHA and EPA while bringing almost ZERO of the Omega-6's which are often much higher in the seeds and nuts than would be ideal. And let's not forget that Cod is very low in Cholesterol and that's exactly why it's a Superfood and one of the best entrées you could choose.[71][96]

40. COD LIVER OIL – 1 Tsp = **40** cal, 90% Vitamin A, 113% Vitamin D3, 888mg OMEGA-3 FATTY ACIDS DHA/EPA, 5%DL SATURATED FAT

As good as Cod is for dinner, Cod Liver Oil is a truly impressive natural dietary supplement. One teaspoon brings 90% RDA amount of Vitamin A as Retinol, 113% Vitamin D3, a difficult Vitamin to get if you are avoiding dairy, and around 888mg of the Omega-3 Fatty Acids DHA and EPA which are proven essential nutrients that promote cardiovascular health. That teaspoon of Cod Liver Oil might taste disgusting, but it brings FOUR critical members of the Big 43 in excellent amounts and it is simply too good for your health to pass up. Because we need to raise the amounts of the Omega-3's versus the Omega-6's found in seeds, nuts and vegetable oils, Cod Liver Oil plays a key role in helping with this in addition to Omega-3 DHA/EPA Supplements.[47]

41. COLLARD GREENS – (cooked) 1 cup (6.7oz) = **49** cal, 308% Vitamin A (as beta-Carotene) 12% Vitamin B2, 12% Vitamin B6, 44% Vitamin B9, 58% Vitamin C, 1045% Vitamin K, 11% Choline, 27% Calcium, 12% Iron, 10% Magnesium, 41% Manganese, 21% FIBER, 177mg OMEGA-3 FATTY ACID ALA, CL: 0.2%

Although my main source has no ORAC Score listing for Collard greens it is expected to be very high due to the huge amount of Vitamin A as Carotenoids. Collard greens are a popular Southern dish and for very good reason; they are loaded with nutrients and are a true Superfood. This is another Brassica (See Cabbage for more details) meaning it is also loaded with sulfur-containing compounds many of which are under investigation for their sundry and powerful health benefits. Collard greens support eye and skin health through their high Carotenoid content, liver detoxification through their Chlorophyll content, lower cholesterol, lower blood pressure, reduce the risk of Colon and Prostate cancer, improve bone health (one of the richest plant sources of Calcium,) and best of all, they are also a true Net Negative Calorie food too and can replace a high calorie low nutritional value side dish and put you on the right track toward better health.[98]

42. CRANBERRIES – 1 cup (3.5oz) = **46** cal, 18% Vitamin C, 16% Manganese, 16% FIBER, ANTHOCYANIDINS, URSOLIC ACID, ORAC Score: 9090, CL: 4.0%[34]

Fresh cranberries might be a bit too tart for most people, but they sure do bring a huge amount of powerful antioxidants. Just as importantly, cranberries are diuretics that prevent water retention and contain a phytonutrient that interferes with the adhesive properties of bacteria allowing them to be flushed away and is the scientifically proven effectiveness of cranberry juice for reducing tooth decay and Urinary Tract Infections. Although cranberry juice is not as potent in antioxidants as the fresh berries, it still scores well (1452) and is highly recommended. Avoid blends and products with additives including those enriched with Vitamin C which will always be synthetic and of dubious quality. But the very best way to cash in on the tremendous antioxidant power of cranberries is to get the dried ones sometimes sold under the name "Craisins." Dried fruits are higher in antioxidant power, the essential nutrients, and phytonutrients than the original fruits.[76]

43. CUCUMBER – (raw) 1 cup (4.7oz) = **16** cal, 19% Vitamin K, 12% Molybdenum, CURCUBATICINS, ORAC Score: 140 (peeled) CL: 1.5%[34]

The Cucumber is the "poster child" of the "melon vines" often called Curcubits which include all forms of squash, Watermelons Cantaloupes, etc. Although they won't impress based on their essential nutrient content, Cucumbers bring Molybdenum mainly because of the way we eat them: raw with the seeds. Studies have shown that the phytonutrients in those seeds help reduce LDL cholesterol and Triglyceride levels, provide potent antioxidant and anti-inflammatory properties (despite the low ORAC Score,) may help prevent and ameliorate Type II Diabetes, protect blood vessel walls and protect blood constituents from oxidative damage, and the unique class of Triterpenoids in them called Curcubaticins have been shown to interfere with cancer cell signaling pathways and may help prevent and even fight cancer. I always advise peeling them because the skins contain a natural insect repellent which is a ketone. These kinds of molecules can be toxic to the kidneys in excess and are also created by the metabolic burning of proteins which is always happening in the body. However, many of the beneficial compounds are highest in the seeds and the skin, so you might choose to leave the skin on them. Finally, Cucumbers are a true Net Negative Calorie food and an excellent health promoting addition to salads,[99]

44. DARK CHOCOLATE – (100% Pure) 4oz. = **560** cal, 108% Iron, 180% Copper, 92% Magnesium, 232% Manganese, 44% Phosphorus, 72% Zinc, 76% FIBER, **180**% SATURATED FAT, CATECHINS, ORAC Score: 49944, CL: 0.9%[34]

Whenever I tell someone that Dark Chocolate is a Superfood, they think I'm crazy. They're right, but not because of my opinion of chocolate. It only has two knocks: 1) It is very high in calories from Saturated Fats, and 2) It is very bitter due to the presence of Tannins, the same compounds that make dark tea bitter. However, it is one of the few easily obtained foods that will bring you at least 100% RDA amounts of Iron AND Magnesium, both of which are difficult to get from natural whole foods. It is also loaded with Catechins which the body is looking for (See Apricots for more details) and finally it has one of the highest ORAC Scores of any true food (only the spices are higher, but you wouldn't sit down to eat a bowl of Oregano.) Because of the high Tannins, eating Dark Chocolate daily is not recommended because it will put a strain on your kidneys, but now and then it can definitely serve to deliver Iron, Magnesium, Zinc, Dietary Fiber, and has been shown in studies to improve mood resulting from improved brain function due to the high antioxidant power of its Catechins. But this isn't candy, that junk is too processed and full of garbage sugar and other chemicals. This is the 100% Pure chocolate you can find in the Baking isle of your grocery store and you can sweeten it with Raw Bee Honey which is also in this list.[57]

45. DRIED PLUMS (Prunes) – 1 cup (pitted, 6.1oz) = **418** cal, 27% Vitamin A (as beta-Carotene) 129% Vitamin K, 19% Vitamin B2, 16% Vitamin B3, 18% Vitamin B6, 24% Copper, 18% Magnesium, 26% Manganese, 12% Phosphorus, 36% Potassium, 49% FIBER, ORAC Score: 8059, GI: 29±4[16][34]

Prunes have the ultimate stigma as "Old Fogey Food" which is why their name has been officially changed to "Dried Plums" which is exactly what they are anyway. Before you scoff at them, take a look at their impressive array of essential nutrients specifically the Potassium and Dietary Fiber content. Despite the high calories they have a very good Glycemic Index because almost all of their sugars must be stopped by the liver to be processed into glucose which slows their arrival into the blood stream and provides the liver with fuel as well. Dried Plums contain concentrated amounts of the same health promoting phytonutrients found in Plums (See Black Plums for more details) and you should consider adding them to your regular dietary regimen.[157]

46. EGG – (hard boiled) 1 large (1.75oz) = **77** cal, 13% Complete Protein, 15% Vitamin B2, 27% Vitamin B7, 25% Choline, 22% Selenium, 18% Iodine, **71%**DV CHOLESTEROL, 8% SATURATED FAT

Eggs are not as evil as they have been portrayed, but they are very high in cholesterol so if you have concerns about that or have been diagnosed with high cholesterol, then you should definitely avoid them until you have that under control. Two eggs for breakfast will bring half of your daily requirement of Choline and we need lots of it and it is very difficult to get from natural whole foods. The yolks are yellow partly due to the presence of beta-Cryptoxanthin, a powerful tetraterpenoid antioxidant very close in molecular structure to beta-Carotene and they are a source of Vitamin A and the health promoting powers of the Carotenoid antioxidants. However, because of the high saturated fat and cholesterol content, they shouldn't be eaten daily. The healthiest preparation is to hard boil them.[100]

47. EGGPLANT – (boiled) 1 cup (3.5oz) = **35** cal, 12% Manganese, 12% FIBER, ORAC Score: 345, CL: 3.5%[34]

Eggplant is one of the few species in its family that is NOT poisonous although it won't win any contests for essential nutrient content or taste, it is a very low calorie food high in mucilage (that's what makes it slimy) that is very good for your digestive tract health. Despite the low ORAC Score the dark purple skin is loaded with a unique anthocyanidin called Nasunin that has been shown to actively protect the membranes of brain cells from oxidative damage (and some folk's brains need all the help they can get!) Eggplant is unusually high in phenolic antioxidants like Chlorogenic Acid which has been shown in studies to be an antimutagen (protects cellular DNA from damage that can lead to cancer.) Chlorogenic Acid also has significant LDL lowering and antiviral properties. One study demonstrated that Eggplant (the juice actually) reduced arterial plaque build up and relaxed blood vessel walls improving circulation. Eggplant is the proof that not all foods need to bring a lot of the Big 43 in order to bring significant amounts of phytonutrients that contribute to better health.[101]

48. FAVA BEANS – (canned) 1 cup (9oz) = **182** cal, 12% Vitamin B3, 21% Vitamin B9, 14% Copper, 14% Iron, 20% Magnesium, 37% Manganese, 20% Phosphorus, 18% Potassium, 11% Zinc, 38% FIBER, CL: 8.7% (est.)

Also known as broad beans, Fava beans are very low calorie for beans meaning they have a high Fiber content (beans like all seeds have very little water in them and are mostly starches, unsaturated fats and Fiber. So whenever any bean is low in calories it is low in starches and fats meaning the bulk of its mass must be Fiber which is simply plant matter that can't be digested. But no two plants have exactly the same forms of Fiber either. Most beans contain a form of Crude Fiber (not water-soluble) that is partially broken down during the digestive process and results in antinutritional (read: Toxic) molecules. This is exactly why many folks suffer from indigestion and gas from eating the other much more common beans. The saving grace of Fava beans is their low calories and the high Dietary Fiber content which has been shown to help lower blood cholesterol and alleviate blood sugar issues. Fava beans make an excellent alternative to the other more popular beans.[102]

49. FIG – 3.5 oz, = **74** cal, 10% FIBER, ORAC Score: 3383, CL: 16.26%[34]

Studies have shown that the phytonutrients in Figs may help with digestion, lower blood pressure, and reduce the risk of Age-Related Macular Degeneration. Studies have also shown that it helps lower blood sugar levels and may help prevent and even ameliorate Type II Diabetes. Fresh figs are low in calories for a fruit and high in antioxidant power and an excellent addition to a healthy diet.[103]

50. FLAX SEED – 2 Tbsp (½ oz) = **75** cal, 19% Vitamin B1, 19% Copper, 13% Magnesium, 15% Manganese, 14% FIBER, 13% Phosphorus, 3190mg Omega-3 Fatty Acid ALA, ORAC Score: 1130, CL: 1.6%[34]

Flax seed has become a craze over the past few decades and it is potentially one of the very best sources of the Omega-3 Fatty Acid ALA – Alpha-Linoleic Acid – which not only has been proven to be a potent anti-inflammatory but is also recognized as an essential nutrient for cardiovascular health. The only two knocks I can find concerning Flax seed are: 1) It is very high in calories, although it doesn't take much to provide a huge dose of ALA, and 2) It has rather low nutritional content of vitamins and minerals. But it does bring a large amount of Dietary Fiber which is necessary for intestinal health and helps lower Cholesterol absorption as well. You can add 2 tablespoons of ground Flax seed to the morning oatmeal and get in on the health benefits of the ALA and the Fiber, and ground Flax seed is also very resilient to heat so it can also be added to the dough of various baked goods and deliver these nutrients in good amounts in those foods as well.[105]

51. GOJI BERRY (Dried) ¼ cup = **100** cal, 140% Vitamin A (as beta-Carotene) 100% Vitamin B2, up to 163% Vitamin C, up to 10% Calcium, 10 to 100% Iron, 25% Potassium, 91% Selenium, 12% FIBER, ORAC Score: 4310[34]

Although the information is for dried Goji berry (and dried fruits have higher concentrations of all nutrients,) there is no denying the health benefits of Goji Berries and they have been a featured food in Traditional Chinese Medicine for thousands of years. Some nutrients can vary greatly from one sample to the next mainly due to environmental conditions of the plants and preparation of the dried berry products, but they are high in nutrients and studies have shown that they can improve immune function, fight certain forms of cancer including skin cancer, improve skin and eye health, stabilize blood sugar, detoxify the liver, improve digestion, improve mood, boost fertility and boost metabolism. No wonder they have been appreciated in China for so long.[106]

52. GRAPES – (red or black) 1 cup (5.3oz) = **104** cal, 27% Vitamin C, 28% Vitamin K, 1% (estimated) Chromium, MYRICETIN, RESVERATROL, QUERCITIN, GALLIC ACID, ORAC Score: 1746 (black) 1637 (red) GI: 59 (black) CL:15.5%[16][34]

Grapes (although raisins are far better) and grape juice, especially dark varieties like Concord, are an excellent source of Chromium for those who don't appreciate Broccoli. I like Broccoli but don't want to eat it every day, so 100% Pure Concord grape juice can provide Chromium every other day of the week. But that's only the beginning of the amazing health benefits of these wonderful little fruits. Dark Grapes contain amongst their many constituents found mainly in their skins, Anthocyanidins, a group of strong flavonoid antioxidants, Myricetin an oddball that is BOTH an antioxidant and a pro-oxidant at the same time: it delivers its typical antioxidant health benefits while also serving as a potent antiviral agent, and last but not least is Resveratrol. This is a stilbenoid similar in properties to Pterostilbene (See Blueberries for more details) and it has been shown to interfere with three key cellular processes that lead to cell death. To coin a phrase it makes all of the cells in your body "Live long and prosper." Is it an "immortality" elixir? Probably not, but it might be the cause of the "French Paradox." Folks in rural France (and other wine producing regions) who sip on their wines daily from childhood have higher average life spans than other communities who do not. Since Resveratrol is found concentrated almost entirely in the grape skins and since wine is made with the grape skins, there may be something to it after all. Avoid daily overindulgence. There is evidence that grapes and their by-products can put a dangerous strain on the kidneys.[50]

53. GRAPE JUICE – (100% Concord) 1 cup (8oz) = **152** cal. 32% Chromium, 6% Magnesium, 8% Potassium, 30% Manganese, ORAC Score: 2389 (100% Pure Concord) CL: 14.2%[34]

Pure Concord grape juice is very nutritious and will bring you much needed Chromium which participates in Insulin signaling pathways and helps blood sugar regulation and metabolism. Chromium is a difficult nutrient to get from natural whole foods and deficiency may be the leading cause of Type II Diabetes worldwide. Getting enough Chromium is a real challenge but it can definitely help those with blood sugar issues and even reduce the risk of Type II Diabetes. Although grapes and their by-products are full of sugar, it is the good kind called "Fructose" which must be stopped and processed by the liver resulting in a slower absorption into the bloodstream. Grapes are high in Tannins so avoid eating too many grapes or drinking the juice on a daily basis. There is evidence that this can put a dangerous strain on the kidneys.[50]

54. GRAPEFRUIT – 1 medium fruit (9oz) = **82** cal, 14% Vitamin A (as Beta-Carotene,) 118% Vitamin C, 14% Vitamin B5, 14% Copper, 10% FIBER, SYNEPHRINE, ORAC Score: 1640, GI: 47±5 (red, canned in juice) CL: 6.9%[16][34]

Grapefruit is actually a hybrid accidentally discovered on the island of Barbados and is a cross between Pomelo and Orange. Like Pomelo it is high in Synephrine; a compound similar to Ephedrine which was very popular in the 1980's as a weight-loss wonder drug until it was banned because a few people took too much and suffered the consequences. While not as potent as Ephedrine, it does stimulate fat burning metabolism and those who begin a calorie restricted diet can definitely benefit from eating grapefruit. But this effect is not just beneficial for losing weight; improving fat burning metabolism can help anyone convert to a leaner healthier body. The Limonoids found in all citrus fruits particularly grapefruit, limes and lemons have been shown in studies to actively prevent cancer cell proliferation and are easily absorbed and persist in the blood stream far longer than most other natural cancer fighting phytonutrients. Limonoids are also being investigated for their ability to lower cholesterol as well. Grapefruit is lower in calories than most other fruits, high in Vitamin C and red and pink varieties bring carotenoids; strong antioxidants and sources of Vitamin A. They are best eaten by letting them fully ripen and then peel and eat like an orange. In other words, resist the temptation to garnish them with processed white cane sugar which is basically toxic.[36]

55. GREEN BEANS – (canned) 1 cup (4.75oz) = **16** cal, 11% Vitamin B9, 65% Vitamin K, 6% Chromium, 13% Manganese, ORAC Score: 290, CL: 0.8%[34]

Green beans are an outstanding Net Negative Calorie Food at just 3.4 calories per ounce. Fresh, raw Green Beans have an ORAC Score of 799, higher than raw carrots, so they do have plenty of antioxidants in them prior to being overcooked at the cannery. Get this wonderful vegetable fresh in the Produce section of your favorite grocery store and either steam them or briefly sauté them to get in on their antioxidant power. Snap beans or "Italian Green Beans" are very similar though not as often available fresh.[107]

56. GREEN PEAS – (canned) 1 cup (6oz) = **118** cal, 192% Molybdenum, 30% FIBER, COUMESTROL, ORAC Score: 120, GI: 25±6 (dried, boiled) CL: 4.2%[16][34]

Although common, Green Peas are truly remarkable. Canned have admittedly been overcooked, but they still bring two days worth of Molybdenum, an essential nutrient required by the body in order for us to be able to put the Sulfur in our foods to use in building and maintaining connective tissues, especially in the joints. A recent study in Mexico demonstrated that 2mg/day of Coumestrol can significantly reduce the risk of some forms of stomach cancer. One cup of Green Peas brings as much as 10mg making them well worth adding to your weekly dietary regimen. Add to that their high Dietary Fiber content and surprisingly low calories and they are a real winner.[70]

57. GUAVA – 1 cup (diced) 5.8oz = **112** cal, 628% Vitamin C, 20% Vitamin B9, 19% Copper, 12% Manganese, 20% Potassium, 36% FIBER, ORAC Score: 1422

This tropical fruit has some rare health benefits. Aside from the usual reducing blood sugar and lowering cholesterol, Guavas have strong antibacterial powers and kill digestive tract worms. Guava has also shown efficacy in treating diarrhea, stomach spasms and hyperactive gut disorders. Only Acerola berry is higher in Vitamin C and Guava is being studied to offer a commercial product that will provide both Dietary Fiber and Antioxidant content. In the meantime, add this amazing fruit to your tropical fruit salad.[163]

58. HONEY (raw, pure) – 1oz = **81** cal, ORAC Score: 130, GI: 69±8 (Clover honey) CL: 81%[16][34]

Make no mistake, Raw Bee Honey is a powerful Functional Food. The complex sugars that comprise the bulk of it and make it resemble fresh engine oil are far superior to plain processed white cane sugar. It might have a very high Glycemic Index, but when compared to the huge percentage of these complex sugars it is actually surprisingly low. The liver has to stop all of these sugars and do chemistry on them to convert them into glucose which can then be released into the blood. This process slows its absorption and release into the blood and the liver cells actually get their energy from doing this chemistry on these complex sugars which it stores as Glycogen. The liver is the only organ in the body whose cells do NOT actually burn sugar for energy; they get their energy from these processes they perform on the raw molecules from our foods. Honey is therefore "liver fuel." But that's only the beginning. Bees don't have refrigerators and keep their honey at ambient temperature, yet it doesn't spoil because it contains traces of natural antifungal and antibacterial compounds of enormous interest to modern science mainly because they are: non-toxic and very effective. When we consume honey, the liver recognizes these compounds and sends them on into the blood stream and they can help prevent and ward off fungal and bacterial infections. Despite the low ORAC Score, raw honey contains: Pinocembrin, Pinostrobin and Chrysin, three powerful flavonoid antioxidants. Pinocembrin has studies showing that it supports enzyme activity and causes apoptosis (programmed cell death) in certain cancer cell lines. Numerous studies have shown that local raw honey can help ameliorate the effects of hay fever because it contains the same pollens that cause the reaction and consuming them helps the person to desensitize to them. Research has shown that raw honey contains the best forms of carbohydrates to be consumed prior to and following strenuous work, exercise or athletic activity. Want more? Studies have shown that the consumption of honey acts as an appetite suppressant and can help those trying to lose weight and it does bring less carbs in superior forms to those in refined white cane sugar because it takes far less to make your food as sweet. Honey replenishes the liver's Glycogen fuel supply before bedtime which will keep the liver from sending an alarm to the brain to wake up and find food in the middle of the night. It also triggers the production of insulin and this triggers the release of Tryptophan in the brain which gets turned into neurotransmitters including melatonin; so a touch of raw honey in warm milk is a definite sleep aid. Sweeten coffee, tea, and breakfast Oatmeal with this very healthy alternative. But don't over do it; Honey is extremely astringent and causes dehydration and is VERY DANGEROUS to babies and toddlers for this reason.[108]

59. HONEYDEW – (diced) 1 cup (6.25oz) = **63** cal, 53% Vitamin C, 12% Potassium, 8% FIBER, ORAC Score: 253, CL: 9%[34]
This is another excellent low calorie melon in the Curcubit family (along with Cucumber and Watermelon, also in this list.) The Carotenoids in Honeydew have been shown in studies to reduce

the risk of cancer, reduce the risk of cardiovascular disease and reduce inflammation while the Dietary Fiber has been shown to help lower cholesterol. For a bland tasting fruit it is surprisingly high in Vitamin C which improves skin health and the immune system.[109]

60. KALE – (raw chopped) ½ cup (1.2oz) = **17** cal, 100% Vitamin A (as beta-Carotene) 68% Vitamin C, 347% Vitamin K, 13% Manganese, LUTEIN, ZEAXANTHIN, CHLOROPHYLL, 5% FIBER, ORAC Score: 1770, CL: 0 (trace)[34]

Kale has the highest amounts of Lutein and Zeaxanthin of any readily available food; two powerful tetraterpenoid antioxidants in a class called Xanthophylls which are yellow colored photosynthetic molecules that all plants possess in their leaves. Both Lutein and Zeaxanthin are found in high concentrations in the human eye, an organ with a very high metabolic rate leading to severe oxidative stress. These antioxidants are appreciated by the cells in the eye and greedily absorbed when available in the blood stream. There has been no conclusive proof from studies linking these two compounds directly to eye health or the prevention or treatment of such maladies as cataracts or Macular Degeneration, but since they are antioxidants and present in very high concentrations in the eye has led most medical professionals to the conclusion that they are significant and can definitely help prevent these vision problems. This is why the leafy greens are a top priority and the added bonus is that they are all loaded with Vitamin K and true Chlorophyll which is the number one liver detoxifier from natural whole foods. And these leafy dark greens are all very low calorie side dishes. Raw is certainly better so add a few leaves of Kale to your lunch salad and get in on its outstanding health benefits.[67]

61. KIWI – 1 cup (6.25oz) = **108** cal, 11% Vitamin B9, 21% FIBER, 273% Vitamin C, 13% Vitamin E, 89% Vitamin K, ORAC: 862, 16% Potassium, 12% Copper, GI:58±7, CL: 9%[16][34]

Kiwis are not just delicious, they have higher Vitamin C content than citrus fruits. Kiwi fruit also brings a lot of Vitamin K, unusual for a fruit, and it is also high in Potassium and Fiber making it one of the most nutritious commonly available fruits.[35]

62. LAMB – (raw, lean cut) 5oz. = **340** cal, 25%DV Complete Protein, 380%DV Vitamin B2, 75%DV Vitamin B12, 40%DV Selenium, 75%DV Zinc, 55%DL SATURATED FAT, **35%DL** CHOLESTEROL

Lamb is an exceptional meat. Though higher in calories than fish and poultry, it more than makes up for this by bringing a lot of Vitamin B2 – Riboflavin and Zinc, difficult essential nutrients to get in sufficient quantities from natural whole foods. Like all meats, Lamb contains Cholesterol, and like all land herbivores it brings a lot of Saturated fat, so for those with high Cholesterol or who are watching their weight, keep the portions small.[74]

63. LEEKS – (cooked) 1 cup (3.5oz) = **32** cal, 29% Vitamin K, 11% Manganese, KAEMPFEROL, ORAC: 569 (raw) CL: 2.1%[34]

Leeks are in the same genus (Allium) as Onions and Garlic. And although they have a milder watery taste, they are still loaded with basic sulfur compounds and antioxidants (see Cabbage and Onions for more details.) A notable flavonoid antioxidant found in significant amounts in Leeks is Kaempferol shown in numerous studies that it protects blood vessel walls from oxidative damage. Although little research has been done with this vegetable, due to the presence of many sulfur-containing compounds and flavonoids Leeks are expected to bring many of the benefits of Onions and the other cruciferous vegetables. More importantly, they are an excellent side dish by themselves or can be added to soups, stews, etc. Researchers are recommending that people should consume 1.25 cups of the Allium family of plants daily for superior health and Leeks are a great way to help increase your regular intake of this important family of edible plants and their powerful and unique phytonutrients.[110]

64. LENTILS – (boiled) 1 cup (7oz) = **230** cal, 90% Vitamin B9, 25% Copper, 37% Iron, 18% Magnesium, 49% Manganese, 21% Potassium, 330% Molybdenum, 17% Zinc, 63% FIBER, ORAC: 7282, GI: 21±7 (dried, boiled) 45 (canned)[16][34]

Wow, these tiny legumes are a true Superfood. Just one cup will almost cover your requirement of Vitamin B9 – Folate, provide over a third of your daily requirement of Iron (more than 3oz of Beef Liver!) half of your requirement of Manganese, and three days worth of Molybdenum while adding to your daily intake of Zinc, Magnesium, and Potassium. They also provide nearly two-thirds of your daily requirement of Dietary Fiber and it is hard to get all 25 grams daily from foods. And finally, Lentils bring over TEN TIMES the antioxidant power of raw carrots. The very high Fiber and Antioxidant content guarantees that Lentils will have a significant impact on lowering cholesterol, lowering blood sugar levels, reducing the risk of cardiovascular disease, and help reduce the risk of many forms of cancer, especially Colon cancer. Lentils are an excellent example of how overcooking beans and similar foods can raise their Glycemic Index considerably.[64]

65. LETTUCE – (Iceberg, shredded) 1 cup (2.5oz) = **10** cal, 22% Vitamin K, 3% FIBER, ORAC Score: 438 – 1532 (depending on the variety) CL: 2.0%[34]

While plain old Iceberg Lettuce is about 95% water, it still brings more than you might expect. Aside from the obvious advantage of being a very low calorie food, it does have some water soluble fiber and almost a fourth of your daily Vitamin K. Most importantly it is filling; making it the definition of a Net Negative Calorie food. Two cups total 20 calories while two cups of potatoes would total about 300. Most people do not realize that Iceberg lettuce has a good ORAC Score of 438 with other varieties scoring a lot higher.

A lunch salad of Lettuce plus additional fresh vegetables like Spinach or Kale brings good health promoting antioxidants and Vitamin K while avoiding lots of trash calories.[111]

66. LIMA BEANS – 1 cup (8.5oz) = **190** cal, 11% Vitamin B6, 30% Vitamin B9, 22% Copper, 24% Iron, 24% Magnesium, 44% Manganese, 300% Molybdenum, 18% Phosphorus, 15% Potassium, 15% Selenium, 10% Zinc, ACE INHIBITOR, 30% FIBER, ORAC Score: 243[34]

One cup of Lima beans can help fulfill your daily requirements of both Iron and Magnesium, two difficult minerals to get for natural whole foods. They are higher in Dietary Fiber and lower in Crude Fiber than most other beans and bring a lot of Molybdenum. Studies have shown that Lima beans have a specific protein that when broken down in our digestive tract yields a substance that acts as a strong Angiotensin Converting Enzyme Inhibitor – the same kinds of compounds that are prescribed to patients suffering from chronic high blood pressure. For those already taking ACE Inhibitors, ask your doctor before loading up on Lima beans. They also possess Alpha-Amylase Inhibiting activity. This prevents the breakdown of complex sugars and starches in the digestive tract into simple sugars that can be absorbed. This means that Lima beans lower the effective calories of all of the rest of the starchy foods in the meal. Want more? Lima beans have been shown in studies to lower blood cholesterol levels, lower blood sugar levels, help protect the liver, protect brain cells from chemical damage, and have shown promise in stopping the growth or breast cancer. Now that should be enough to get them on the menu![112]

67. LOW SODIUM ORIGINAL V-8 BRAND VEGETABLE JUICE – 12oz glass = **67** cal, 34% Potassium, 180% Vitamin C, 12% FIBER, ORAC Score: 548 (generic vegetable juice)[34]

This is an excellent low calorie drink that brings plenty of health benefits. Primarily it is the only way to get a handle on all of that Potassium (3500mg) that is needed daily. The Low Sodium version is made to taste salty with Potassium salts rather than Sodium salt and it takes more Potassium salt to maintain its original flavor. That is excellent news because it is loaded with the Potassium that we desperately need.[73]

68. MANGO – 1 cup (5.8oz) = **99** cal, MANGIFERIN, ORAC Score: 1300, GI: 51±3[16][34]

Don't underestimate the power of orange colored fruits. They indicate the presence of flavonoids and carotenoids which are powerful antioxidants and some can be converted into Vitamin A. Mangos are alone in their genus (Mangifera indica) because they are actually a natural genetic accident and came from a species of Bouea, a small genus of rare tropical fruit trees found in Southeast Asia. Mangos have a unique phytonutrient called Mangiferin along with many other health promoting compounds. Mangos have been shown to possess anti-allergenic, antibacterial, anti-inflammatory, and antioxidant properties. Mangoes help lower cholesterol, lower blood sugar levels, alleviate gastric ulcers, protect against cell damage from harmful radiation (a relatively rare and significant power) and have shown promise in fighting certain forms of Colon, Breast and Prostate cancer cell lines. Add some of this tasty tropical fruit to your weekly diet and you will reap many healthy rewards.[113]

69. MILK – (Whole, 3.25% fat) 1 cup (8oz) = **146** cal, 9% Complete Protein, 24% Vitamin D3, 26% Vitamin B2, 28% Calcium, 23% SATURATED FAT, **8%**DV CHOLESTEROL

Whole milk is still the most readily available source of both Vitamin D3 and Calcium in natural forms for most people. Skim milk loses a lot of Vitamin D3 in particular as the fat is removed. Whole milk and dairy products also bring some much needed Complete Protein as well. For those with lactose intolerance, there only a few high calcium plants: Broccoli, Bok Choy and Collard Greens.[116]

70. MUSSELS –(steamed) 4oz = **195** cal, 53% Complete Protein, 25% Vitamin C, 23% Vitamin B1, 28% Vitamin B2, 17% Vitamin B3, 11% Vitamin B5, 21% Vitamin B9, 453% Vitamin B12, 43% Iron, 11% Magnesium, 385% Manganese, 32% Phosphorus, 10% Potassium, 145% Selenium, 17% Sodium, 20% Zinc, 5% SATURATED FAT, 21%DL CHOLESTEROL

Ever wonder why the Japanese have the healthiest society? Their diet is mainly low calorie vegetables and sea food and Mussels are a good example bringing huge amounts of Manganese, Selenium and Vitamin B12 along with a long list of other essential nutrients in good quantities including Iron, Zinc and Complete Protein.[117]

71. NAPA CABBAGE – (cooked) 1 cup (3.8oz) = 13 cal, 12% Vitamin B9, 11% Manganese, CHLOROPHYLL, CL: 0 (trace)

Napa cabbage is a great alternative vegetable for cooking into stews because it is much sweeter than most of the other varieties and has just 3.3 calories per ounce, only Watercress and Pickles (also in this list) have fewer calories per ounce. It can fill you up on a healthy leafy green that brings Folate and Chlorophyll (See Arugula for more details) rather than trash calories.[118]

72. NEW ZEALAND SPINACH – (raw) 1 cup (2oz) = **8** cal, 49% Vitamin A (as beta-Carotene) 9% Vitamin B6, 28% Vitamin C, 18% Manganese, CL: 0 (trace)

Although I can't find the ORAC Score for this up and coming vegetable, it is expected to be high with such a high amount of Carotenoids in it (the Vitamin A.) This is another very low calorie food that is said to taste sweeter than most other raw green leafy vegetables and is suitable for raw salads. It has a long history as a holistic medicinal plant used to treat inflammatory problems as well as women's hormonal issues such as symptoms of menopause. Studies have shown that New Zealand Spinach has a significant ability to lower cholesterol and inhibit the formation of fat cells. Another study showed that it also inhibits alpha-Amylase, alpha-

Glucosidase, and Aldose Reductase. These enzymes are involved in breaking down carbohydrates in the intestines and by inhibiting them, fewer starches are converted into sugars reducing the total caloric intake of the entire meal. It might be hard to find, but it is certainly an excellent addition to your diet especially if you are trying to lose a few extra pounds or just want to stay trim.[119]

73. MUNG BEANS – 1 cup (7.1oz) – **212** cal, 22% Vitamin B1, 80% Vitamin B9, 16% Copper, 16% Iron, 24% Magnesium, 30% Manganese, 20% Phosphorus, 15% Potassium, 11% Zinc, 61% FIBER, CL: 2.9%

This is another Net Negative Calorie bean (29.7cal/oz) that brings a lot of Folate and Dietary Fiber. Both of these nutrients when obtained from natural whole foods have been linked to reduced risk of cancer and Mung Beans can replace any of the inferior popular beans like Navy, Pinto or Kidney beans.[165]

74. OATS – (precooked) ½ cup (1.4oz) = **150** cal, 15% Chromium, 74% Manganese, 64% Molybdenum, 26% Vitamin B7, 17% FIBER, 5400mg BETA-GLUCANS, ORAC Score: 1708, GI: 59±4, CL: 58.9%[16][34][155]

Oats, specifically old-fashioned whole grain oatmeal are a real winner and the only thing you should eat for breakfast. Although high in calories, we do need them in the morning so we have fuel to start the day and they bring several essential nutrients, a good start towards getting your fill of Dietary Fiber and most importantly, they are one of the few plants that contain the all-important Beta-Glucans (See Button Mushrooms for more details.) You can mix it with water and put it in the fridge over night and make "raw" oatmeal which retains more of these very powerful phytonutrients. You can empty the spice rack into it adding flavorful antioxidant powerhouses like Cinnamon, Ground Vanilla Bean, Nutmeg, or Allspice along with seeds, nuts, and fruits and turn it into a tasty breakfast cereal bringing a whole smorgasbord of nutrients.[68]

75. OKRA – (raw) 1 cup (3.5oz) = **31** cal, 13% Vitamin B1, 11% Vitamin B6, 22% Vitamin B9, 35% Vitamin C, 66% Vitamin K, 14% Magnesium, 50% Manganese, 13% FIBER, CL: 2.5%

Although my source does not provide the ORAC Score for Okra, it is expected to be high due to beta-Carotene, Lutein and other antioxidant constituents. Okra brings more nutrients than most people expect. It is an excellent source of Vitamin B9 – Folate, one of the more difficult B Vitamins to get from natural whole foods. Studies have shown that a high Folate natural foods diet will significantly reduce the risk of cancer although researchers have yet to discover the mechanism behind this effect and they also note that supplements do not have the same measurable effect on lowering the risk of cancer. Okra is also an excellent source of Vitamin K, Magnesium (very difficult to get natural whole foods) and Manganese. Foods high in Manganese have been shown to help alleviate many women's hormonal imbalance issues. Okra is high in Myricetin and studies have shown that this substance can substantially lower blood sugar levels although the mechanism is again unknown at this time. The specific type of Lectins in Okra have been shown in preliminary studies to kill up to 74% and to halt the growth of 63% of the breast cancer cells exposed to them. Okra has a reputation as a mood enhancer and as the "plant Viagra" possibly due to its unusual forms of complex sugars which appear to have a strong effect on relaxing the blood vessels to improve circulation. Such foods have an enormous impact on the brain which is full of tiny restricted blood vessels and capillaries and the brain cells have an extremely high metabolic rate and need good blood flow. Add to all of this a good source of Dietary fiber and mucilage (See Eggplant for more details) and Okra is an excellent choice for improved colon health. Okra does contain oxalates which can accumulate as Kidney and urinary tract stones. Like all good things, Okra should only be consumed in moderation; perhaps just once a week.[120]

76. OLIVES (and 77. OLIVE OIL) – (black, canned) ½ cup (2.4oz) = **77** cal, 19% Copper, 12% Iron, 7% FIBER, KAEMPFEROL, HYDROXYTYROSOL, ANTHOCYANIDINS, QUERCETIN, OLEANOLIC ACID, APIGENIN, FERULIC ACID, GALLIC ACID, ORAC Score: 1010 – 3130, CL: 0 (trace)[34]

Olives, black or green, are truly amazing. There is a lot of ongoing research into the health promoting powers of their dozens of unique phytonutrients called Phenylethanoids. Olives are powerful medicine for the human body and Extra Virgin Olive oil, also loaded with many of these phytonutrients is one of only a few oils I recommend, especially for home-made salad dressing. Oleanolic Acid is a powerful triterpenoid nutritional fatty acid that has been shown in research to have liver protective properties as well as anti-inflammatory, antiviral and antitumor properties (slows, halts the growth or even shrinks cancer tumors.) Hydroxytyrosol, one of those Phenylethanoids unique to Olives, has been linked to reduced risk of certain forms of cancer and may prevent bone loss as well. Methylated Gallic Acid yields Methyl Gallate which has been shown to be very potent in selectively targeting and killing certain brain cancer cell lines. This is not to say that Olives and Olive oil can "cure" cancer, but synthetic compounds similar to those found in them are under investigation for their potential as cancer treatments. Ranging from one and a half to over four times the antioxidant power of the same weight of raw carrots, toss a cup of these unusual fruits into your stew and reap the excellent benefits for your heart and overall cardiovascular health while adding a whole slew of powerful cancer stoppers too. (See Apples, Blueberries, Celery, Leeks, and Onions, for more details on the other phytonutrients found in Olives.)[114][164]

78. ONIONS – (chopped) 1 cup (7.4oz) **92** cal, 27% Vitamin B7, 16% Vitamin B6, 27% Vitamin B7, 15% Vitamin C, 16%

Copper, 14% Manganese, 11% Phosphorus, 11% FIBER, SULFUR, FISETIN, QUERCETIN, FERULIC ACID, ORAC Score: 600 – 1500 (depending on the variety) CL: 4.7%[34]

Onions are loaded with health promoting phytonutrients and are an excellent source of basic sulfur compounds. The body needs this mineral in order to construct connective tissues especially for the joints. Glucosamine Chondroitin is a joint support supplement precisely because both of these compounds contain Sulfur (See Cabbage for more details.) Onions also contain very powerful antioxidants which comes as a surprise to many people. And of great importance to this entire discussion is the fact that scientists have only recently discovered a new flavonoid in them called Fisetin. This underscores the fact that all natural plants contain hundreds of individual compounds that we know about and probably as many that we have yet to isolate and identify. Yet, the human body is well aware of them, the liver recognizes them and passes them on through to the blood stream and cells throughout the body happily absorb them and put them to work improving their health and performance. Onions are one of the richest sources of Quercetin which has many health benefits (See Apple for more details.) Ferulic Acid, while very common and found in virtually all plants, is bound to the proteins in their cell walls and has a rather low bioavailability. Onions give it up easily and it has been shown to neutralize the oxidants that do damage to DNA and may indeed help reduce the risk of many forms of cancer. Raw chopped onions create a detrimental compound which in small amounts causes no trouble and is neutralized after a few minutes, but a brief sauté or boil also gets rid of it and provides you with a bounty of antioxidants and sulfur-containing compounds.[121]

79. OYSTERS – (canned, boiled) 2oz. = **38** cal, 25% Complete Protein, 180% Vitamin B12, 124% Copper, 340% Zinc, 294mg OMEGA-3 FATTY ACIDS DHA/EPA, 1% SATURATED FAT, **10**%DL CHOLESTEROL

Like all animal foods, Oysters bring some Cholesterol which is a component of virtually all animal cell membranes. Plants on the other hand don't have cholesterol in them. The good news is that you only need ONE ounce of oysters, and canned boiled oysters will do, to provide you with a great dose of Vitamin B12 – critical for proper brain function, and no other food comes close to the amount of Zinc in Oysters, more than enough to cover it for the day.[53]

80. PAPAYA – 5oz = **50** cal, 112% Vitamin C, 13% Vitamin B9, 8% FIBER, PAPAIN, ORAC: 300, GI: 56±6, CL: 7.8%[16][34]

Like all fruits, Papaya is loaded with antioxidants despite the deceptively low ORAC Score. But it is the Papain found in this delicious fruit that contributes to its scientifically proven health benefits including the ability to assist in the breakdown of proteins in the digestive tract, making more amino acids available to be absorbed and used by the rest of the body. And Papaya has been shown to reduce the risk of Colon cancer, so try to add this fruit rich in antioxidants, flavonoids, and sundry health benefits to your weekly tropical fruit salad.[115]

81. PARMESAN CHEESE (hard or grated) 3oz. – **330** cal, 60% Complete protein, 100% Calcium, **69**%DL SATURATED FAT, **18**% CHOLESTEROL

All natural cheeses bring saturated fat and cholesterol. It comes from the dairy cream in which the fungi cultures are grown. Most fat free cheeses lose a lot of their natural nutritional content from the processing that removes the fat. Luckily it only takes three ounces of Parmesan (or Romano, they are very similar) to bring you 100% of your daily requirement of Calcium in a pure and natural form that the body can readily absorb. I apply some to my lunch salad as well as my tomato sauce based entrées to get this natural Calcium rather than take supplements which are always inferior and a potentially dangerous way to get Calcium. Because of the high Saturated Fat in Parmesan and other natural Cheeses, look to sea food as the entrée for the day, most fish and shellfish are very low in Saturated Fat.[44]

82. PEANUTS (and Peanut Butter) 3oz. = **495** cal, 57% Vitamin B3, 51% Vitamin B7, 39% Vitamin E, 33% Magnesium, 63% Manganese, 15% Zinc, **10**%DL SATURATED FAT, ORAC Score: 3166 (kernels.) Peanut butter: ORAC Score: 3432, GI: 23±3, CL: 14%[16][34]

Peanuts are not true nuts, but actually legumes more closely related to Green peas than Pecans. But they do have "nut-like" properties including the fact that they are loaded with fats. Peanuts have been shown in numerous studies to improve heart and cardiovascular health due to the nutritional fatty acids in them as well as the very powerful array of antioxidants and the specific essential nutrients they bring, but only in moderation![33]

83. PECANS – 3oz. = **597** cal, 24% Vitamin B1, 48% Copper, 12% Iron, 27% Magnesium, 165% Manganese, 24% Phosphorus, 27% Zinc, 33% FIBER, 27% SATURATED FAT, ORAC Score: 17,940, CL: 4.3%[34]

Did you know that 3 ounces of Pecans bring the same amount of antioxidant power as nearly 5 POUNDS of raw carrots? In fact, that would be almost 876 calories worth of carrots meaning that ounce for ounce and calorie for calorie, Pecans actually have a higher antioxidant DENSITY than raw carrots. Unfortunately, it doesn't take much to fill you up on excessive amounts of calories, but they do bring Magnesium and Zinc, both difficult to fulfill during the day and a third of your daily requirement of Dietary Fiber. If you limit your dinner to the entrée plus two Net Negative Calorie side dishes like Green Beans and Beets, desert can be a cup of low fat Yogurt with a few ounces of sliced Kiwis and Pecans, a personal favorite of mine.[122]

84. PICKLES – 3.1 cal/oz (See Cucumbers and Vinegar for more details) Cal/oz, GI and CL vary depending on added sugars. Pickles are another outstanding Net Negative Calorie Food. But you will be hard-pressed to find a jar of them not laced with that infernal Yellow #5. Pickled cucumbers bring the phytonutrients of the Cucumbers, plus the antioxidant and holistic medicinal powers of the spices and the Vinegar. Instead of munching bags full of greasy, salty, starchy potato chips, I enjoy a jar of "Bread and Butter Chips" style pickles instead. Can't find a good pickle product without that cancer-causing Yellow #5 in it? Make your own: Slice your cucumbers (they pickle faster when sliced) and place them in a clean jar. 2) Fill half way with White vinegar, 3) Add about ½ teaspoon of Turmeric powder (this is the original healthy formula for making them yellow) 1 Tbsp of dill weed, and any other spices you might like (I add 1 Tbsp each of minced garlic, oregano and black pepper) 4) Seal the jar and shake it up, 5) Finish filling the jar with Red Wine Vinegar to get in on the powerful phytonutrients of grapes and the sweeter taste (See Grapes for more details,) 6) Throw it into the back of the fridge for a few months, 7) Serve your own healthy delicious pickles.[99][124]

85. PINEAPPLE - (chunks) 1 cup (5.8oz) = **83** cal, 11% Vitamin B1, 11% Vitamin B6, 105% Vitamin C, 20% Copper, 67% Manganese, 8% FIBER, BROMELAIN, ORAC Score: 943, GI: 66±7, 43 – 55 (canned in juice) CL: 9.8%[16][34]

This unusual member of the Bromeliad family brings a bounty of health benefits primarily due to the high essential nutrient content, its powerful antioxidants and the Bromelain. Like Papain found in Papayas, this compound assists the digestion of proteins and Pineapples have also been linked to improving the immune system. They are, like many fruits, rather low calorie and while the juice does bring the same constituents, the actual fruit brings far higher concentrations of them.[125]

86. PISTACHIOS – 3oz. = **480** cal. 48% Vitamin B1, 54% Vitamin B6, 57% Copper, 54% Manganese, 36% FIBER, 24%DL SATURATED FAT, ORAC Score: 7675. CL: 9.2%[34]

Pistachios are another great nut. Aside from being quite tasty they bring a lot of Vitamin B6 – Pyridoxine, which is one of the toughest B Vitamins to fulfill during the course of the day because no single food brings 100% RDA amounts in a convenient serving size. This does make B6 one of my "Watchout Nutrients" that might be best addressed with a supplement. They also bring plenty of Vitamin B1, a huge amount of antioxidants and Dietary Fiber. Pistachios do bring Saturated Fat (like all nuts.)[56]

87. POLLOCK – (raw) 4 oz. = **103** cal, 44% Complete Protein, 12% Vitamin B2, 20% Vitamin B3, 60% Vitamin B12, 13% Choline, 20% Magnesium, 24% Phosphorus, 12% Potassium, 60% Selenium. 496mg OMEGA-3 FATTY ACIDS DHA and EPA, 1%DL SATURATED FAT, **28%DL CHOLESTEROL**

Pollock easily makes this list because it has the distinction of being a meat with extremely low saturated fat: just 1% Daily Limit in 4 ounces, and it is a Net Negative Calorie food at 25.8 cal/oz. It also brings nearly 100%DV of the Omega-3 Fatty Acids DHA and EPA. Because of the high water content, they do shrink when cooked, but the caloric and nutritional content won't change.[126]

88. POMEGRANATE – 1 cup (6.1oz) = **144** cal, 16% Vitamin B9, 30% Vitamin C, 36% Vitamin K, 12% Potassium, 28% FIBER, PUNICIC ACID, ORAC Score:4479[34]

Pomegranates have been a popular fruit since ancient times. They contain a class of unique compounds called Punicalagins which are extremely powerful antioxidants giving the fruit or the juice three times more antioxidant strength than red wine or green tea. Punicic Acid is a unique form of Conjugated Linoleic Acid which is a well known anti-inflammatory nutritional fatty acid. Studies have shown that regular consumption of Pomegranates or their juice helps lower blood pressure, improves circulation, lowers LDL cholesterol levels, lowers the risk of certain forms of cancer including breast and prostate cancer, helps alleviate Benign Prostate Hyperplasia (enlarged prostate) lowers the risk of heart disease, improves cognitive function and memory and can ease symptoms of arthritis. They might not cure anything, but those powerful unique compounds have been shown that they will provide a wide spectrum of significant health benefits.[127]

89. PORK – (chops, top loin, trimmed) 5oz = **276** cal, 75% Complete Protein, 60% Vitamin B1, 15% Vitamin B2, 60% Vitamin B3, 10% Vitamin B5, 50% Vitamin B6, 15% Vitamin B12, 19% Choline, 32% Phosphorus, 16% Zinc, 85% Selenium, **23**% SATURATED FAT, **34**% CHOLESTEROL

Well trimmed choice cuts of Pork are actually quite nutritious in many ways starting with a very high density of quality Complete Protein. Add to that excellent amounts of Vitamin B1, B3, B6 (a hard one to get from natural whole foods) as well as Selenium and quality fresh pork is an excellent choice for the dinner entrée, but bacon, sausage, hot dogs, etc are to be AVOIDED.[151]

90. PUMPKIN – (canned) 1 cup (8.6oz) = **83** cal, 763% Vitamin A (as beta-Carotene) 17% Vitamin C, 13% Vitamin E, 49% Vitamin K, 13% Copper, 19% Iron, 14% Magnesium, 18% Manganese, 14% Potassium, 28% FIBER, ORAC Score: 483 (raw) GI:66±4, CL: 5.2%[16][34]

Most people don't think of Pumpkin Pie filling (100% pure and unsweetened) as a Superfood, but the definition of Superfood is: "Brings 100%DV of at least one essential nutrient in a convenient portion size" and 763% of your daily requirement of Vitamin A per cup sure fits the bill. Pumpkin is loaded with antioxidants starting with all of that beta-Carotene and it has a respectable amount of Vitamin E for a fruit which is also a valuable antioxidant. One cup of Pumpkin is just 83 calories and brings almost as much Iron as 3 ounces of Beef Liver which also brings 231mg of Cholesterol (78% Daily Limit) while Pumpkin brings ZERO. Those 7 grams of Dietary Fiber are also very respectable and the reason Pumpkin is so filling and good at lowering cholesterol. Cook it into soups and stews or add a little black pepper and garlic to the canned pumpkin and heat it up for an excellent low calorie side dish that brings a lot of Nutrients, Fiber and Antioxidants and relatively few calories to the meal.[128]

91. PUMPKIN SEEDS – (roasted) 4oz. = **500** cal, 40% Copper, 72% Magnesium, 28% Manganese, 28% Potassium, 76% Zinc, **20%** SATURATED FAT, 24% FIBER, CL: 0 (trace)

If Pumpkin is good for you, Pumpkin Seeds might be even better. Pumpkin seeds like all seeds and nuts are loaded with excellent nutrition. Also they have slightly fewer calories per ounce than most other seeds and nuts which raises their Nutrient DENSITY per calorie. For those who do not wish to indulge in Oysters, by far the least expensive and easiest way to get your daily Zinc is about 5 ounces of Pumpkin seeds which will also bring almost all of your daily requirement of Magnesium (another very difficult mineral to get,) but be aware, because that is also about 625 calories and 24% of your Daily Limit of Saturated Fat.[55]

92. RAISINS – 3.5oz = **300** cal, 16% Copper, 12% (estimated) Chromium, 10% Iron, 15% Manganese, 10% Phosphorus, 21% Potassium, ORAC Score: 3406, GI: 64±11[16][34]

There is little doubt that grapes are a significant source of nutrients since raisins now bring their entries in this list up to three (with one more to go!) Raisins are confounding to say the least. Many folks list them as "excellent sources" of so many nutrients (See Grapes for more details) and they may well be the ONLY sources of some of the more difficult ones to get like Chromium for some people. But most full nutrient analysis reports I have seen indicate that they either have no Chromium, or the food wasn't tested for it. But since grape juice and wine are good sources, then dark grapes and raisins must have Chromium in them. It won't evaporate or decompose; it's a metal. Since grapes and grape juice can put a strain on the kidneys, raisins could also cause trouble.[129]

93. SALMON – (raw fillet) 4oz. = **171** cal, 30% Complete Protein, 44% Vitamin B3, 37% Vitamin B5, 15% Vitamin B7, 144% Vitamin B12, 148% Vitamin D3, 48% Selenium, 1500 to 2300mg Omega-3 Fatty Acids DHA/EPA, ASTAXANTHIN, 6%DL SATURATED FAT, 24%DL CHOLESTEROL

Salmon is one of the heavier species of "oily" fish and has a bit more saturated fat than some of the others, but it is still lower than most land animals and is one of the healthiest meats on Earth. It is loaded with Vitamins B12 and D3 and brings about half of your daily requirement of Selenium, not only needed by the Thyroid gland but also a powerful antioxidant in its own right. And Salmon are also loaded with the Omega-3 Fatty Acids DHA and EPA which have been proven to support heart and blood vessel health. Even though the ORAC Score for Salmon is low, it does contain Astaxanthin, which is what makes their flesh red, an antioxidant that is SIX THOUSAND TIMES more potent than Vitamin C. The fish get it from eating certain species of red algae, so wild-caught Salmon is greatly preferred.[42]

94. SARDINES – (canned) 4oz = **233** cal, 56% Complete Protein, 168% Vitamin B12, 76% Vitamin D3, 44% Calcium, 56% Phosphorus, 84% Selenium, 17% Choline, 1650mg OMEGA-3 FATTY ACIDS DHA and EPA, 8%DL SATURATED FAT, **52**%DL CHOLESTEROL

Every once in a while I used to get a craving for a can of Sardines in Mustard sauce. It is critical to listen to your cravings because scientists are starting to suspect that this is how the brain makes us consume foods that contain essential nutrients that are severely DEPLETED in the body. You can bet these cravings were related to any one or more of the many essential nutrients that Sardines bring including Vitamin B12, Vitamin D3, Calcium, Selenium and plenty of the Omega-3 Fatty Acids DHA and EPA. But be aware: they bring a lot of Cholesterol too.[62]

95. SCALLOPS – (raw) 4 oz. = **77** cal, 47% Complete Protein, 102% Vitamin B12, 30% Choline, 90% Iodine, 69% Phosphorus, 45% Selenium, 16% Zinc, 220mg OMEGA-3 FATTY ACIDS DHA and EPA, **50**% SODIUM, 1.2%DL SATURATED FAT, 16%DL CHOLESTEROL

It can't be an accident that I have always liked the lower calorie sea foods since I was a kid growing up in South Florida and Scallops were a favorite and they are tied with Cod fish as the lowest calorie meat on Earth at 19.3 calories per ounce. Aside from having such a low amount of calories which is a boon to help make room for some of the other higher calorie Superfoods in this list, they also bring almost no Saturated Fat and relatively little Cholesterol in a four ounce serving. Like most sea foods they are high in Sodium (they use it to counter the Sodium in the seawater so they don't dehydrate through osmosis) but Scallops are rich in Iodine, in a far better form than that in Iodized Salt, Choline which is another essential nutrient that is very difficult to get from natural whole foods, and bring a large amount of Phosphorus which is linked to detoxification of the body. The 220mg of DHA and EPA Omega-3's is respectable (although most other sea foods in this list bring more) and proven essential nutrients for the heart and vascular system. A full dose of Vitamin B12 completes the picture, along with the Choline, as a valuable "brain food."[130]

96. SESAME SEED BUTTER (TAHINI) – 1oz, **167** cal, 23% Vitamin B1, 12% Calcium, 23% Copper, 14% Iron, 20% Manganese, 20% Phosphorus, 10% FIBER, 11%DL SATURATED FAT

A casual glance at the nutrient content of Sesame Seed Butter might not impress you very much, but there is much more going on in these health promoting seeds than just the Big 43. Studies have shown that Sesame Seeds actually lower the amount of Sodium in relation to the amount of Potassium in the blood which is IDEAL for improving electrolytic balance, osmotic pressure throughout the body and reducing blood pressure. And this brings up another key to the general argument of this book; it is still a mystery as to how the Sesame Seeds actually do this. Tahini is made the same way as peanut butter but instead of peanuts they just mash up whole Sesame seeds and the result is a spread that brings all of their remarkable health benefits.[131]

97. SHRIMP – 4oz. = **135** cal, 52% Complete Protein, 11% Vitamin A (as Retinol) 19% Vitamin B3, 12% Vitamin B5, 16% Vitamin B6, 78% Vitamin B12, 17% Vitamin E, 17% Choline, 32% Copper, 31% Iodine, 50% Phosphorus, 102% Selenium, 17% Zinc, 375mg Omega-3 Fatty Acids DHA/EPA, **72%**DL CHOLESTEROL, 2%DL SATURATED FAT, ASTAXANTHIN

Although rather high is Cholesterol, Shrimp are a great low calorie entrée that will bring your entire daily requirement of Selenium along with many other essential nutrients. Some Shrimp do have Astaxanthin in them, one of the most powerful antioxidants known, but it varies not only by species, but also from one individual shrimp to the next. Raw red fleshed shrimp are the most likely to have it in them since the compound is a deep crimson red. Shrimp can help with many hard to get Vitamins like B5, B6, as well as Choline and even Vitamin E which is almost unheard of in animal meat products.[132]

98. SOUR CREAM – 1oz. = **57** cal, 16%DL SATURATED FAT, 6%DL CHOLESTEROL, CL: 3.5%

This is certainly not to be confused with a Superfood or even necessarily a Functional food, so why is it in this list? It is a far superior food to the one it can replace: mayonnaise and its kin, the creamy dips and salad dressings. Sour Cream is a dairy product that will at least bring a little Calcium and Phosphorus but most importantly, it will not block those critical B Vitamins and is a far superior choice. You can make your own healthy dips, Tuna, Turkey or Chicken Salad and even salad dressing by mixing some into the Oil and Vinegar dressing.[133]

99. SPINACH – (raw) 1 cup(1.1oz) = **7** cal, 15% Vitamin B9, 181% Vitamin K, 3% FIBER, ORAC Score: 1513, CL: 0.4%[34]

Spinach in any form raw or cooked or even canned is available year round in most grocery stores and is an excellent source of natural Vitamin K and brings very good antioxidant power as well. It might not be at the top of your list of most desirable foods to eat, but it is not as bad as its name makes it sound and it is incredibly low in calories and high in Chlorophyll too (See Arugula for more details.)[66]

100. SPIRULINA – (dried) 1 cup (4oz) = **325** cal. 65% Protein,

178% Vitamin B1, 242% Vitamin B2, 72% Vitamin B3, 177% Iron, 55% Magnesium, 44% Potassium, **342%** Copper, 106% Manganese, 16% FIBER, 15%DL SATURATED FAT, CL: 3.1%
Spirulina is loaded with protein although it is technically not the complete kind, it does bring a good dose of the nine essential amino acids. Four ounces brings significant amounts of many important nutrients including Vitamins B1, B2, and B3 as well as Iron, Magnesium, Manganese and Potassium but 4 ounces will also bring too much Copper, so it should only be consumed in much smaller quantities to make sure that averages out to 100% per day.[58]

101. STRAWBERRIES – 1 cup (5oz) = **46** cal, 113% Vitamin C, 24% Manganese, 10% FIBER, ANTHOCYANIDINS, ORAC Score: 4302, GI: 40±7, CL: 4.9%[16][34]

Strawberries are another fruit very commonly found in grocery stores. Most people choose to pass on them due to the "seeds" stuck to the skin, but those are actually the fruits, the strawberry itself is nothing but a swollen stem loaded up with sugar and nutrients like the Anthocyanidins which are powerful antioxidants with some amazing health benefits (See Blueberries for more details.) And don't scoff at its other nutritional offerings like Dietary Fiber, plenty of Vitamin C, and a very low GI for a fruit.[134]

102. SUNFLOWER SEED KERNELS – 3oz. (kernels) = **490** cal, 30% Vitamin B3, 60% Vitamin B5, 33% Vitamin B6, 51% Vitamin B9, 111% Vitamin E, 96% Phosphorus, 78% Copper, 18% Iron, 27% Magnesium, 90% Manganese, 96% Selenium, 21% Potassium, 30% Zinc, **22%**DL SATURATED FAT, 30% FIBER, CL: 2.7%,

If any food in this list deserves to be called a Superfood, it is Sunflower Seed Kernels. Just 3 ounces will provide you with your full daily requirements of Vitamin E, Phosphorus, Manganese and Selenium. That's FOUR members of the Big 43 in one sitting, so while they bring calories, they also knock out a lot of our nutritional requirements and help with Vitamins B5 and B6, Iron, Magnesium, Potassium, Copper, Manganese, Zinc and Fiber. Sunflower Seeds are rich in Omega-6 Fatty Acids which have been shown to help lower cholesterol and have strong anti-inflammatory properties that help prevent and alleviate the symptoms of arthritis and some cardiovascular diseases. A great alternative that has the same nutritional value is Sunflower Seed Butter, a spread similar to Peanut Butter that is a very nutritious substitute.[32][71]

103. SWEET POTATOES – (baked with skin) 1 cup (7oz) = **180** cal, 769% Vitamin A (as beta-Carotene) 14% Vitamin B1, 12% Vitamin B2, 15% Vitamin B3, 18% Vitamin B5, 29% Vitamin B6, 29% Vitamin B7, 16% Copper, 14% Magnesium, 50% Manganese, 11% Phosphorus, 27% Potassium, 26% FIBER, ORAC: 2115, GI: 70±6(avg.) CL: 13.5%[16][34]

The biggest surprise for me was the low calories. In fact, since they have less than 30 cal/oz, they are in my Net Negative Calorie foods list. The greatest power of Sweet Potatoes is the fact that they hold on to much of their antioxidant potential when baked with the skin on (the ORAC Score is for exactly this preparation) and also have the lowest Glycemic Index score of 44 when boiled for 30 minutes or less with the skin. Sweet potatoes deliver an enormous amount of Vitamin A as beta-Carotene which is a powerful antioxidant (no mysteries there) and are also a great source of Dietary Fiber.[136]

104. SWISS CHARD – (raw, chopped) 1 cup (6.2oz) = **35** cal, 60% Vitamin A, 12% Vitamin B2, 42% Vitamin C, 22% Vitamin E, 636% Vitamin K, 10% Calcium, 12% Choline, 32% Copper, 36% Magnesium, 25% Manganese, 20% Potassium, 22% Iron, 13% FIBER, BETALAINS, CHLOROPHYLL, ORAC Score: 1108, CL: 1%[34]

The above paragraph of nutrient contents alone should indicate the health benefits of this leafy vegetable. But a closer look reveals that Swiss Chard is a true Superfood. Significant amounts of Calcium, Vitamin E and Choline are RARE in leafy greens and 1 cup has as much Iron as 3 ounces of Beef Liver without the ton of Cholesterol and only 35 calories making it a true Net Negative Calorie food as well. It is an obvious choice to trade the 78%DL of Cholesterol in the Beef Liver for the 13%DV of Dietary Fiber in Swiss Chard to get the same amount of Iron. Throw in a good amount of Magnesium and Potassium and plenty of antioxidants and Swiss Chard is a clear winner. All leafy vegetables bring Chlorophyll (See Arugula for more details) but the red colors in the leaves are caused by Betalains (See Beets for more details.) Studies have shown no surprises: Swiss chard lowers blood sugar levels, lowers blood pressure (that's the Potassium at work,) lowers cholesterol, and reduces the risk of Type II diabetes, cardiovascular disease and cancer.[137]

105. SWISS CHEESE – (natural) 3oz. = **318** cal, 45% Complete Protein, 66% Calcium, 24% Zinc. **75%** SATURATED FAT, **27%** CHOLESTEROL, CL: 1.3%

Just 3 ounces of this delicious cheese provide much needed Complete Protein, Calcium and some much needed Zinc. If you are trying to avoid the boiled canned Oysters, Swiss Cheese can definitely help you try to fulfill your daily requirement for this critical mineral. However, go easy on the natural unprocessed cheeses. While much higher in nutritional content than cheeses that have had the fat processed out of them, they do bring a lot of saturated fat and cholesterol.[45]

106. TANGERINE – 1 cup (6.9oz) = **103** cal, 27% Vitamin A (as beta-Carotene) 87% Vitamin C, 9% Potassium, 14% FIBER, ORAC: 1627, GI: 47±2 (Mandarins, canned in juice)[16][34]

Like the other citrus fruits Mandarins and Tangerines (they are distinct) contain Limonoids which have been shown to be very beneficial (See Grapefruit for more details.) In addition, Tangerines in particular contain a phytonutrient called Nobiletin, which might actually have better activity than the Synephrine in Grapefruit; it stimulates fat burning metabolism and also prevents the addition of new fat into the fat cells. Although Lemons and Limes have the highest concentrations of the valuable Limonoids, no one can eat them, but Tangerines and Grapefruits are a great way to get them plus Vitamin C and their unique and powerful phytonutrients.[138]

107. TEFF – (cooked) 1 cup (8.9oz) = **255** cal, 31% Vitamin B1, 11% Vitamin B3, 12% Vitamin B6, 11% Vitamin B9

Teff is a grain that has at least 25% less calories per ounce than any of the others. In fact, it is the lowest calorie grain on Earth (that I can find anyway.) Although relatively rare and unknown at this time, I do think its heyday is coming as people try to find ways to lower their trash calorie intake. Just one slice of plain store-bought white bread brings about 70 calories, that's 140 calories for the bread of a sandwich. With Teff bread that would come out to about 50 calories instead. The flour is available from some specialty vendors online and I plan to give it a try. Saving 90 cal. per sandwich is the kind of savings that can be reinvested in some true Superfoods like Sunflower Seed Kernels and it makes baking with Teff well worth the effort.

108. TOMATO – (raw diced) 1 cup (6.3oz) = **32** cal, 30% Vitamin A (as beta-Carotene,) 24% Vitamin B7, 38% Vitamin C, 16% Vitamin K, 4% Chromium, 12% Copper, 20% Molybdenum, 12% Potassium, 9% FIBER, LYCOPENE, ORAC Score: 387(raw) – 548 (freshly cooked) CL: 2.6%[34]

Tomatoes might not bring much in the way of essential nutrients but they more than make up for it in Lycopene. This powerful antioxidant which is about 40 TIMES more potent than Vitamin C and what makes them red has numerous studies including human trials demonstrating a wide range of seemingly miraculous health benefits. The health benefits of Lycopene sound almost too good to be true, but researchers have shown that Lycopene: 1) Is a powerful anti-inflammatory and may help ease arthritis. 2) Helps prevent and combat several forms of cancer including breast, prostate, and others, 3) Prevents and fights cataracts and blocks actions in the cells of the eye that lead to Macular Degeneration, 4) Alleviates neuropathic pain caused by nerve damage in the soft tissues or other difficult to combat forms of neurological pain like phantom limb pain of amputees, 5) Prevents and even corrects many forms of neurological damage including but not limited to the damage caused by Monosodium Glutamate (MSG,) seizures, Alzheimer's Disease, etc, 6) Linked to the prevention and correction of many forms of cardiovascular disease including coronary heart disease, myocardial ischemia, atherosclerosis, etc, 7) Helps reduce oxidative stress in the bones (its power as an antioxidant shines here) which can help keep the bones from becoming weak and brittle.[156] Unfortunately, studies done with processed Lycopene supplements have shown no conclusive results. All of this evidence was collected from clinical trials of people consuming Tomatoes and other Lycopene-rich foods. Added bonus: cooking them makes the Lycopene even stronger, but only when eaten fresh. Once the tomato sauce cools, the Lycopene is depleted, so store bought tomato sauce products are out and home-made sauce is definitely on the menu. Added bonus: they have a relatively low CL – Carb Load which means they will have a good estimated Glycemic Index of about 10 to 30 for home-made sauce (and much lower raw.)[140]

109. TUNA – (light, canned in water) 5oz. = **162** cal, 21% Choline, 70% Complete Protein, 83% Vitamin B3, 50% Vitamin B6, 400mg OMEGA-3 FATTY ACIDS DHA and EPA, 2.5%DL SATURATED FAT, **15%** CHOLESTEROL

One little can of chunk light tuna in water brings a lot of essential nutrients. It brings a good dose of Vitamin B3 and B6 which are very hard to get from natural whole foods. Try to avoid making Tuna fish salad with mayonnaise which is on the "black list" of foods that are really bad for you. Instead use Olive Oil and Sour Cream. Added bonus; Tuna Fish brings an excellent amount of Complete Protein versus its content of saturated fat (2.5% Daily Limit in a 5oz serving) and cholesterol compared to most other animal meat products and is one of my Top Recommended Superfoods for that reason alone, but another great benefit comes from the 80%DV of the Omega-3 Fatty Acids DHA and EPA.[61]

110. TURKEY – (light meat, skinless, boneless) 6oz = **264** cal, 100% Complete Protein, 60% Vitamin B3, 50% Vitamin B6, 25% Choline, 78% Selenium, 9%DL SATURATED FAT, **36%DL** CHOLESTEROL

Baked or Rotisserie Turkey breast is a great source of Complete Protein, although the method of preparation can dramatically affect the caloric content due mainly to the presence of the skin. Like chicken, Turkeys store a lot of saturated fat in the skin and the connective tissues between it and the muscles. Cholesterol content can also vary widely if the skin is present or not and be sure to check the labels on things like packaged sandwich meats (that they use ONLY the lean meat) especially for preservatives and artificial colors like Nitrites which are dangerous, damaging OXIDANTS and TOXIC to the liver. Although the serving size is higher than any other meat in this list, lean Turkey breast is low in Saturated Fat (9% Daily Limit for a 6oz serving) and calories and an easy way to get 100% of your daily requirement of Complete Protein and plenty of Vitamin B3, B6, and Selenium.[141]

111. TURNIPS – (boiled, diced) 1 cup (5.5oz) = **34** cal, 30% Vitamin C, 12% FIBER, CL: 3%

Turnips are an excellent low calorie alternative to plain high starch, high calorie, high GI potatoes. For that reason alone, they are on the menu. In fact, you can make mashed turnips instead of potatoes and use them in just about as many ways as potatoes although the precise recipes might have to be altered slightly to accommodate them. Turnips have a bit of an unusual flavor which takes a little getting used to, but they are very well worth the effort and add to your daily Vitamin C and Dietary Fiber totals.

112. VEAL – (shank, lean cut, raw) 4oz = **120** cal, 44% Complete Protein, 18% Vitamin B2, 43% Vitamin B3, 15% Vitamin B5, 25% Vitamin B6, 26% Vitamin B12, 22% Phosphorus, 10% Potassium, 13% Selenium, 31% Zinc, 4%DL SATURATED FAT, **28%** CHOLESTEROL.

Very lean cuts of Veal are surprisingly low in saturated fats (4% Daily Limit in 4oz) and calories and a good source of Complete Protein. Like all meats Veal will bring some cholesterol and is often not the most economical meat available, but for the low calories and the excellent spread of nutrients particularly the B Vitamins and the Zinc, it is well worth it.[143]

113. VINEGAR (Red Wine or Apple Cider) – 1oz = 0 to 4 cal. This is the fourth entry for Grapes and their by-products and that should tell you that grapes have enormous health benefits (See Grapes for more details.) Apple Cider vinegar has had much more study than Red Wine vinegar and both bring the phytonutrients found in the original fruits, but the health benefits of Vinegar itself are of interest as well. When a person drinks ½ glass of wine, the liver steps in and stops the alcohol, or more precisely Ethanol, and converts it into Vinegar, or more precisely Ethanoic Acid. Rather than poison the liver with alcohol, just give it the vinegar it truly needs. The liver uses the Acetyl group of the acid in countless metabolic processes and releases it into the bloodstream to act as a pH buffer helping to keep the blood pH correct and making it more resistant to change. This helps osmotic pressure, fluid, and electrolyte balance as well. Studies have shown that vinegar lowers blood pressure, lowers blood sugar and improves insulin sensitivity, and lowers cholesterol all of which in turn reduces the risk of cardiovascular disease. Therefore, Olive Oil and Red Wine Vinegar salad dressing is the only truly healthy choice.[124]

114. WALNUTS – (kernels) 1oz. = **183** cal, 19% Vitamin B7, 22% Copper, 48% Manganese, 8% FIBER, 2600mg OMEGA-3 FATTY ACID ALA, 11,000mg Omega-6 Fatty Acids, 9%DL SATURATED FAT, ORAC Score: 13,541[34]

Walnuts, despite having very little actual Vitamin E in them, still have a very high ORAC Score, so they are loaded up with other powerful antioxidants. They are an excellent source of Omega-3 Fatty Acid, but it is the plant Omega-3 – Alpha-Linoleic Acid. While also very good for you, it might not be able to replace the need for the animal Omega-3's DHA and EPA. Walnuts are delicious and nutritious, but are really high in calories. A good way to add them to your regular diet is to toss an ounce of them into the morning oatmeal from time to time. Like most plant foods that bring a lot of ALA, they also bring a huge amount of polyunsaturated fats and the Omega-6 Fatty Acids found in those fats. These are also very good for your health, but most health professionals are advocating keeping the ratio at no more than five times the Omega-6's to the Omega-3's with 2 to 1 being ideal. Walnuts like many seeds and nuts are around 5 times as many O6FA's versus the O3FA Alpha-Linoleic Acid. This ratio is something that the fish can help fix with their high O3FA content in the needed forms DHA and EPA while bringing much less Saturated Fat and no Omega-6's.[30][71]

115. WATERCRESS – (raw, chopped) 1 cup (1.2oz) = **3.7** cal, 22% Vitamin A (as beta-Carotene) 24% Vitamin C, 106% Vitamin K, 1% FIBER, CL: 0 (trace)

Watercress is the King of the Net Negative Calorie Foods at just 3.7 calories per cup. It may not dazzle in nutrient content, but it has a higher DENSITY of Vitamin K per calorie than even the well known very low calorie greens like Spinach and Kale. You can definitely add it to soups, stews, salads, and so on as an excellent way to increase the portion size while adding almost no extra calories and fulfilling your daily requirement of Vitamin K. To give you an idea of what it means to bring just 3 calories per ounce, you would have to eat over 41 POUNDS of Watercress to reach 2,000 calories for the day. Watercress and the other very low calorie vegetables are a good way to create room for the high calorie Superfoods like the seeds and nuts.[144]

116. WATERMELON – (diced) 1 cup (5.4oz) **46** cal, 16% Vitamin C, LYCOPENE, ORAC Score: 142, GI: 60 – 80 (depends on variety and ripeness) CL: 6.2%[16][34]

Watermelon makes the grade as an excellent Functional Food that provides simple sugars and powerful antioxidants like Lycopene while still being a relatively low calorie food. Most people do not realize that most natural whole fruits, even Watermelon, actually help reduce the risk of Type II Diabetes. Watermelon is a rich source of Lycopene, a powerful tetraterpenoid antioxidant similar to beta-Carotene, but it is about 70% stronger in antioxidant power. Although the body cannot convert it into Vitamin A, it has one of the longest lists of verified health benefits of any compound listed in this book (See Tomato for more details.) So start adding delicious low calorie Watermelon to your diet and remember: "The redder; the better," because Lycopene is a deep red compound and is what makes this fruit's pulp red.[145]

117. WHEAT GERM – ½ cup (2.5oz). = **250** cal, 87% Vitamin B1, 45% Vitamin B6, 50% Vitamin B9, 42% Magnesium, 60% Phosphorus, 60% Zinc, 80% Selenium, **468**% Manganese, 30% FIBER, CL: 38.6% (est.)

The Wheat Germ is the nugget of nutrients within the whole wheat kernel that provides the nutrients for the wheat embryo to begin growing and emerge from the seed. It should come as no surprise that it is loaded with nutrients that are good for our health too. The easiest way to sneak it into your daily eating regimen is in the morning oatmeal and I add several tablespoons into it two days a week. That gives you a very good start on your daily intake of Vitamin B9, Selenium and Zinc although admittedly it also brings a bit too much Manganese which is why it should be limited to this amount just two days a week.[43]

118. YAMS – (boiled, cubes) 1 cup (4.8oz) = **158** cal, 16% Vitamin B6, 27% Vitamin C, 10% Copper, 25% Manganese, 26% Potassium, 21% FIBER, GI: 35±5 (boiled) CL: 23.6%[16]

While they are certainly not a Superfood, they are a far superior choice to regular old high calorie potatoes. Yams contain complex carbohydrates and Fiber which give them a much lower Glycemic Index – the break down in the digestive tract results in fewer sugars that take longer to enter the blood stream. Their GI goes way up the longer they are cooked including canned products which are often overcooked. Yams contain Diosgenin, a studied phytoestrogen that can help with women's hormonal issues and has been linked to possibly reducing the risk of osteoporosis as well. Yams, like Beets and Turnips are an excellent healthy alternative to potatoes and other Nonfunctional high calorie/low nutritional value foods.[146]

119. YEAST EXTRACT SPREAD ("Marmite" or "Vegemite") 1oz. = **44** cal, 181% Vitamin B1, 235% Vitamin B2, and 136% Vitamin B3, 18% Vitamin B6, 71% Vitamin B9, 13% Magnesium, 21% Potassium, **42**% SODIUM.

Yeast Extract Spread, available as the commercial brand names "Marmite" or "Vegemite" is probably the number one Superfood in this entire list. Ounce for ounce and calorie for calorie it has the highest nutrient density of Vitamin B1 – Thiamine, B2 – Riboflavin, B3 – Niacin, and Vitamin B9 – Folate of any food. The extract itself tastes horrific which is why these products add a ton of spices to try to cover that up and it is admittedly an "acquired" taste which is politically correct code for: horrific (the spices fail to cover it up very well!) Two ways to sneak it into your daily diet is to stir some into the morning oatmeal or into soups and stews, but do this after the food comes off the stove so you won't destroy those valuable B Vitamins. For those who consider it an edible dietary supplement of these FOUR critical B Vitamins, just slather it on 100% Whole Wheat local-bakery-made bread or toast. Although I have not been able to verify it, Yeast Extract Spread could contain Beta-Glucans which are a "fungi thing" and other yeast products do have these health promoting compounds (See Button Mushrooms.)[147]

120. YOGURT– (Organic, whole milk) 1 cup (8.6oz) = **149** cal, 17% Complete Protein, 20% Vitamin B2, 10% Vitamin B5, 15% Vitamin B12, 30% Calcium, 47% Iodine, 23% Phosphorus, 11% Potassium, 10% Zinc, **26**%DL SATURATED FAT, **11**%DL CHOLESTEROL

Yogurt, especially organic – made from grass-fed cow's milk, is an excellent source of Calcium and Iodine. Reduced fat products are a bit too processed for my liking and lose some of their nutritional content, but they are lower in calories and are worth considering. Adding your own fresh fruits and nuts is a great way to add their health promoting power to the yogurt. A personal favorite is Kiwi and Pecan (that's a ton of Vitamin C and a blast of antioxidants, by the way.) Another advantage of Calcium-rich foods is that they improve satiety – the feeling of being full which means they tend to reduce the amount of calories you would normally consume along with them. This is why your Yogurt "dessert" should actually come BEFORE the rest of the meal – it really works.[46]

121. ZUCCHINI – (boiled) 1 cup (6.3oz) = **29** cal, 40% Vitamin A (as beta-Carotene) 14% Vitamin C, 10% Magnesium, 13% Potassium, 10% FIBER, ORAC Score: 180, CL: 1.7%[34]

Zucchini along with yellow squash are both excellent Net Negative Calorie foods and like Cucumbers bring the added bonus that we normally eat the seeds as well as the pulp. This greatly increases their nutritional value. This is another food with a deceptively low ORAC Score, but it does bring a lot of the Carotenoids which have been shown to reduce the risk of cardiovascular disease and cancer. Don't disregard the Magnesium and Potassium either. Those two are hard to get from natural whole foods and can help you piece them together from real foods rather than supplements which are always inferior and potentially dangerous. Personally, I greatly prefer Yellow squash over Zucchini, but it is delicious when breaded with corn flour and fried which is admittedly not the healthiest food on Earth. But frying them in health promoting oils like Olive Oil, Sesame Seed Oil or Coconut Oil turns a normally evil food into an excellent opportunity to get in on the amazing health benefits of these oils.[148]

CONCLUSION

That's 121 foods and many are superfoods that can provide all of the Big 43 Essential Nutrients from the best possible sources: natural whole foods. If all of your weekly dietary choices came from this list while taking care not to exceed 2,000 calories per day, and staying under 100% Daily Limits of both Saturated Fat and Cholesterol, and not exceeding 100% RDA amounts for the minerals and oil-soluble vitamins: that would be what Doctor's call a "Proper Diet."

Aside from the changes to the daily requirements of the essential nine amino acids in recent years, the main obstacle is knowing how much of each of them you need daily, and how much of them are actually present in your foods. And it is important to remember that chronic illness and genetic predisposition can also spur the need for the conditionally essential amino acids as well.

DOING THE MATH FOR THE ESSENTIAL AMINO ACIDS
This is yet another issue that complicates matters regarding the nine essential amino acids; you have to figure out how much you need of each on a daily basis.

The RDA's of the nine essential amino acids that I have provided are the amounts published by the U.S. government (the Food and Drug Administration) and other agencies like the World Health Organization have published different amounts. Histidine has an RDA of "19mg/kg" meaning you need 19mg (milligrams) per kg (Kilogram) of body weight. One Kg = 2.2 pounds (roughly) so a 180lb individual weighs: 180 ÷ 2.2 = 81.8kg. And he needs 19mg per kg: 81.8 x 19 = 1554mg of Histidine per day. Therefore:

EACH ESSENTIAL AMINO ACID DAILY REQUIREMENT
1. Get your weight in kg: pounds ÷ 2.2
2. Multiply that by the RDA amount of the amino acid.

Another convenient way to get all nine quickly is like this:

FIGURE OUT ALL NINE EASILY
1. Figure out your requirement of Tryptophan.
2. Tryptophan amount times 3 = Histidine.
3. Tryptophan times 3.8 = Isoleucine, and the combination of Methionine + Cysteine
4. Tryptophan times 4 = Threonine
5. Tryptophan times 5 = Valine
6. Tryptophan times 6.6 = Phenylalanine + Tyrosine
7. Tryptophan times 7.6 = Lysine
8. Tryptophan times 8.4 = Leucine

It should be clear that Lysine is needed in quite a large quantity daily and yet it is usually deficient in plant proteins and one of the main reasons why I define "Complete Protein" as any animal meat which have much larger quantities of it and can much more easily fulfill the daily requirement without forcing you to eat much higher quantities of proteins which are dirty burning fuels that result in higher concentrations and worse forms of metabolic waste by-products in the cells and tissues than burning carbohydrates.
EXAMPLE:

A 200lb person weighs 90.9kg (200 ÷ 2.2) and will need:
Tryptophan: 90.9 x 5(mg/kg) = 454mg
Histidine: 454 x 3 = 1,362mg
Isoleucine: 454 x 3.8 = 1725mg
Methionine + Cysteine: 454 x 3.8 = 1725mg

Threonine: 454 x 4 = 1816mg
Valine: 454 x 5 = 2270mg
Phenylalanine + Tyrosine = 454 x 6.6 = 2996mg
Lysine = 454 x 7.6 = 3450mg
Leucine: 454 x 8.4 = 3813mg

All of these amounts should be considered rough estimates and you do not have to adhere to them as strict requirements. The same could be said for all of the Big 43. The idea is to make sure that you do not fall way short day after day, or get far too much of any of them day after day

QUANTITIES OF THE NINE ESSENTIAL AMINO ACIDS

Rather than list each of the nine essential amino acids one by one, I'll list each food one by one and the amounts of each amino acid they bring per ounce unless otherwise specified. The top row of each table lists the amino acids by the first three letters of their names. The value below them is the amount in milligrams found in the specified weight of the food. The value under that is the multiple of the amount of Tryptophan which will therefore be 1.00. A white box for these multiples indicates that the value is close to the proper proportion according to the RDA's established above. A light gray box indicates that it is below ideal and a medium gray box indicates a serious shortage. For those with multiple medium gray boxes, the worst is indicated in dark gray. A plus sign "+" indicates a surplus of the amino acid above the ideal proportion. In Almonds, the combination of Methionine + Cysteine is well short of ideal as is the amount of Lysine which is to be expected in plant foods. Leucine, Threonine and Valine while short of the ideal amounts are tolerable. The amounts of Isoleucine and Histidine are very close to ideal and the total for Phenylalanine and Tyrosine is well above ideal. The ratio of Methionine to Cysteine should be 2.5-to-1 and Phenylalanine to Tyrosine should be 1-to-1. Severe discrepancies are indicated by an asterisk in the boxes where they occur. In Almonds, both pairs are far from ideal ratios.

1, ALMONDS – (roasted) 1oz = 167 cal, **6.2g Protein**, 6%DL SATURATED FAT

Iso	His	Leu	Lys	Met	Phe	Thr	Try	Val
201	172	428	175	137	488	197	55.7	233
3.60	3.08	7.68	3.14	2.46*	+8.76*	3.54	1.00	4.18

Although the seeds and nuts are excellent sources of protein, one ounce of Almonds contains about 1/3 of the Lysine of most animal meats and about 1/3 of the Methionine as well. Also the ideal protein should provide about twice the amount of Methionine as Cysteine and about equal amounts of Phenylalanine as Tyrosine. The rest of the essential amino acids are present in good amounts.

2. ATLANTIC MACKEREL (raw, fillet) – 1oz = 57.5 cal, **5.2g Protein**, 13%DL SATURATED FAT, 5%DL CHOLESTEROL

Iso	His	Leu	Lys	Met	Phe	Thr	Try	Val
240	153	423	478	209	379	228	58.2	268
4.12	2.62	7.26	+8.2	3.60	6.51	3.91	1.00	4.60

This is the first of the animal meat products and it brings typical amounts of the essential amino acids and in proper proportions. There should be about 2.5 times the amount of Methionine to Cysteine and Phenylalanine should be roughly the same amount as the Tyrosine and both pairs are close to these ideal ratios in Atlantic Mackerel.

3. BEEF, SIRLOIN (raw, lean only) – 1oz = 49.6 cal, **8.6g Protein,** 3%DL SATURATED FAT, 5%DL CHOLESTEROL

Iso	His	Leu	Lys	Met	Phe	Thr	Try	Val
392	275	686	729	336	616	344	56.6	428
4.15	2.91	7.27	7.72	3.56	6.53	3.64	0.60	4.53

Beef is very deficient in Tryptophan which skews the rest of the values. It is the low amount of Tryptophan that keeps Beef from being a very good source of Complete Protein; just average. And you should not rely on it heavily. Poultry is a better source of Tryptophan and the rest of the essential amino acids. Sirloin steak or the leanest Sirloin hamburger is a very good source of Zinc and can be included once in a while to help you get enough of this critical mineral for the day.[149]

4. BEEF LIVER (raw) – 1oz = 37.8 cal, **5.7g Protein,** 2%DL SATURATED FAT, 26%DL CHOLESTEROL

Iso	His	Leu	Lys	Met	Phe	Thr	Try	Val
271	176	535	450	257	530	243	73.6	353
3.68	2.39	7.27	6.11	3.49*	+7.20*	3.30	1.00	4.80

Beef liver is a rich source of true Complete Protein, but it is very high in saturated fat and cholesterol. As such you should consume no more than 3 ounces in any meal and because of the very high copper content, this should be restricted to about twice a week.[48]

5. BLACK BEANS (canned) – 1oz = 25.6 cal, **1.7g Protein,** 7.76% FIBER

Iso	His	Leu	Lys	Met	Phe	Thr	Try	Val
74.5	47	135	116	44.0	138.6	71.1	19.9	88.2
3.74	2.36	6.78	5.83	2.21*	6.98*	3.57	1.00	4.43

Black Beans have also been included to serve as an example of the poor forms of proteins in plants. Many seeds and nuts actually bring quite a bit of protein. Black beans bring typical amounts for beans and the expected incorrect proportions of Methionine to Cysteine and Phenylalanine to Tyrosine as well as the shortages of Lysine and Methionine are also clearly visible in the analysis.

6. CHICKEN (raw, breast, skinless) – 1oz = 30.8 cal, **6.5g Protein,** 0.5%DL SATURATED FAT, 5%DL CHOLESTEROL

Iso	His	Leu	Lys	Met	Phe	Thr	Try	Val
201	147	485	549	261.9	475	273	75.6	321
2.65	1.94	6.41	7.26	3.46	6.28	3.61	1.00	4.24

The poultry meats are outstanding sources of Complete Protein, and unusually high in Tryptophan. Because of this, the relative amounts have been given a little more leeway than usual. This makes Chicken a great source of the essential amino acids that still come up with white boxes and it is still a fairly good source of Leucine even though it is somewhat deficient.[94]

7. CHICKEN LIVER (raw) – 1oz = 32.5 cal, **4.7g Protein**, 2%DL
   SATURATED FAT, 32%DL CHOLESTEROL

Iso	His	Leu	Lys	Met	Phe	Thr	Try	Val
142	147	423	373	197	414	203	49.3	279
2.88	2.98	8.58	7.56	4.00*	+8.39*	4.11	1.00	+5.6

Chicken Liver is a Superfood for the many vitamins and minerals it brings in significant quantities but it is also one of the highest sources of saturated fats and cholesterol of any animal product. This is unfortunate because it also brings a well balanced array of the nine essential amino acids as well. Just 3 ounces brings 100% of your Daily Limit of Cholesterol and should be considered the maximum amount for any single meal and no other sources of cholesterol should be consumed on that day.[95]

8. CLAMS (canned) – 1oz = 41.4 cal, **7.2g Protein**, 0.5%DL
   SATURATED FAT, 6%DL CHOLESTEROL

Iso	His	Leu	Lys	Met	Phe	Thr	Try	Val
311	137	503	534	254.8	485	308	80.1	312
3.88	1.71	6.28	6.67	3.18*	6.05	3.84	1.00	3.89

Clams are a rich source of Tryptophan – only milk and the other dairy products are higher – and this tends to skew some of the other essential amino acid amounts which was taken into account in the gray boxes. Clams are one of the richest sources of Vitamin B12 as well as Iron. Because the Tryptophan is needed by the brain cells for constructing neurotransmitters and the B12 is also needed by the brain, Clams are not just a Superfood, they are a "Super Brain Food."[54]

9. COD (Atlantic, raw) – 1oz = 23.0 cal, **5.0g Protein**, 0.18%DL
   SATURATED FAT, 4%DL CHOLESTEROL

Iso	His	Leu	Lys	Met	Phe	Thr	Try	Val
230	147	405	458	201	363	219	55.7	257
4.13	2.64	7.27	8.2+	3.60*	6.52	3.93	1.00	4.61

Cod has an excellent array of the nine essential amino acids in some of the best proportions and amounts of any protein. It's also a Net Negative Calorie food (less than 30cal/oz) with incredibly low amounts of Saturated Fat and very low Cholesterol for any meat making it an ideal choice for getting your Complete Protein and Iodine for the day.[96]

10. EGG (1 large, hard-boiled) – ≈1.75oz = 77.5 cal, **6.3g Protein**,
   8%DL SATURATED FAT, 71%DL CHOLESTEROL

Iso	His	Leu	Lys	Met	Phe	Thr	Try	Val
343	149	538	452	342	591	302	76.5	384
4.5+	1.94	7.03	5.91	4.47+	7.72+	3.94	1.00	5.02

It is a shame that eggs bring so much cholesterol because they do have an excellent array of the nine essential amino acids. Because of the high cholesterol you should stick to hard boiled eggs and no more than two every other day.[100]

11. GOAT (raw) – 1oz = 30.5 cal, **5.8g Protein**, 1% SATURATED FAT, 5%DL CHOLESTEROL

Iso	His	Leu	Lys	Met	Phe	Thr	Try	Val
292	120	481	429	223	377	275	85.7	309
4.5+	1.84	7.4	6.6	3.44	5.8+	4.23	0.76	4.75

Most Americans are not interested in goat meat, but it is very popular in many Caribbean islands. Until you have tried Curry Goat, don't knock it. Goat meat is very rich in Tryptophan: far higher than Turkey with its reputation of causing drowsiness due to its "high" Tryptophan content. Once this is taken into account, the rest of the amino acids actually show up in very respectable ratios. Very lean cuts are low in calories, only missing the Net Negative Calorie foods list by ½ calorie per ounce and are also surprisingly low in Saturated fat and Cholesterol.[158]

12. HAM (deli, sliced, unflavored, avg. 11% Fat) – 1oz = 45.6 cal, **4.6g Protein**, 4%DL SATURATED FAT, 5% CHOLESTEROL

Iso	His	Leu	Lys	Met	Phe	Thr	Try	Val
160	134	276	311	133	257	156	43.4	188
3.68	3.08	6.35	7.16	3.09	5.92	3.59	1.00	4.33

Sliced deli ham is not the worst source of Complete Protein but many essential amino acids are lower than they should be. It does bring 22,9mg Choline/oz (4%DV.) Because it has a high water content, the amount of protein per ounce is a bit lacking but it is actually about average for what is found in some sea foods.[152]

13. LAMB (trimmed, domestic) – 1oz = 68 cal, **4.9g Protein**, 11%DL SATURATED FAT, 7%DL CHOLESTEROL

Iso	His	Leu	Lys	Met	Phe	Thr	Try	Val
237	156	382	434	184	365	210	57.4	265
4.13	2.72	6.65	7.56	3.21	6.36	3.6+	1.00	4.61

Aside from being an excellent source of Vitamins B3, B12 as well as Zinc, Lamb is an excellent source of Complete Protein but it does bring saturated fat, cholesterol and calories like most land animals and you should watch the portion sizes accordingly.

14. MILK (Whole) – 8oz cup **= 146** cal, **7.9g Protein**, 23%DL SATURATED FAT, 8%DL CHOLESTEROL

Iso	His	Leu	Lys	Met	Phe	Thr	Try	Val
403	183	647	342	224	730	349	183	468
4.5+	2.03	7.18	3.80	2.49	8.11+	3.87	2.0+	5.2

Milk and all dairy products are extremely high in Tryptophan, no other source of Complete Protein has higher concentrations. Given that, the ratios were treated as if it had 90mg/oz and four of the eight other essential amino acids still fell short, and two came up in significant excess. The levels are significantly different because the Milk is intended for young calves and not adults. All this suggests is that dairy should not be your principle source of Complete Protein and the high levels of Tryptophan are excellent for brain health.[116]

15. MUSSELS (steamed) – 1oz = 48.2 cal, **6.7g Protein**, 1%DL SATURATED FAT, 5%DL CHOLESTEROL

Iso	His	Leu	Lys	Met	Phe	Thr	Try	Val
290	128	469	498	237	452	287	74.8	291
3.87	1.71	6.27	6.65	3.17	6.04	3.83	1.00	3.89

Mussels are another excellent source of the nine essential amino acids and are also high in Tryptophan which skews their ratios. They are a great source of Iron, Selenium and plenty of Vitamin B12. If there is one knock on Mussels it is that they also loaded with Manganese: too much to eat them daily.[117]

16. OYSTERS (canned, boiled) – 1oz = 19.3 cal, **2.0g Protein**, 1%DL SATURATED FAT, 5%DL CHOLESTEROL

Iso	His	Leu	Lys	Met	Phe	Thr	Try	Val
86.0	38.1	139	148	70.5	134	85.1	22.1	86.2
3.89	1.71	6.24	6.7	3.19	6.06	3.85	1.00	3.9

These are below the typical amounts per ounce for the mollusks. Because of their ratios and low caloric value, oysters are a good source of the essential nine amino acids although they are slightly deficient in Histidine and Methionine. However, you can overdose on Zinc and Copper trying to get your 100% daily allowance of Complete Protein exclusively from Oysters raw or cooked.[53]

17. PARMESAN CHEESE – 1oz = 110cal, **10.0g Protein**, 23%DL SATURATED FAT, 6%DL CHOLESTEROL

Iso	His	Leu	Lys	Met	Phe	Thr	Try	Val
530	387	967	926	333	1097	369	135	687
3.92	2.86	7.16	6.85	2.47*	8.12+	2.73	1.00	5.08

Parmesan (and Romano which is very similar) Cheese is the first cheese in this list and it is a true Superfood when it comes to what it brings. Just 3 ounces will bring ALL 1000mg of Calcium you need for the day and it will also bring about 90% of each of the nine essential amino acids required by the average 200lb person. It is very high in Tryptophan like all dairy products making it a rich source of this critical amino acid needed by the brain. If there is a knock in its Complete Protein profile, it is deficient in Cysteine which we can make for ourselves anyway.[44]

18. POLLOCK (raw) – 1oz = 25.8 cal, **5.4g Protein**, 0.22%DL SATURATED FAT, 7%DL CHOLESTEROL

Iso	His	Leu	Lys	Met	Phe	Thr	Try	Val
251	160	442	500	219	397	239	61	281
4.11	2.62	7.24	8.19	3.59	6.50	3.92	1.00	4.60

Pollock is another fish that is hard to beat in terms of low calories and very low saturated fat content while bringing a good array of the essential nine amino acids in their proper proportions. A 200lb person would need about 7.5 ounces to get his daily requirement of Tryptophan which would only bring 2%DL of Saturated Fat, about 52%DL Cholesterol, and just 193 calories.[126]

19. PORK (chops, top loin, boneless) – 1oz = 55.2 cal, **7.4g Protein**, 4%DL SATURATED FAT, 7%DL CHOLESTEROL

Iso	His	Leu	Lys	Met	Phe	Thr	Try	Val
367	322	634	691	291	596	334	78.4	389
4.7+	4.1+	8.08	8.8+	3.71	7.60+	4.26	1.00	4.96

Believe it or not, Pork is one of the better sources of Complete Protein. The ratios of the nine essential amino acids are very close with only a few going slightly over the expected norms and not by much. Lean cuts are also low in saturated fat and cholesterol.[151]

20. SALMON (raw) – 1oz = 42.8 Cal, **6.1g Protein**, 1%DL SATURATED FAT, 6%DL CHOLESTEROL

Iso	His	Leu	Lys	Met	Phe	Thr	Try	Val
272	140	426	493	305	415	277	86.8	314
3.13	1.61	4.90	5.67	3.51	4.78	3.19	1.00	3.61

Salmon is another Superfood fish that brings Vitamin B3, B12 and Selenium and plenty of the Omega-3 Fatty Acids DHA and EPA. It is relatively low in Saturated fat and Cholesterol compared to land animal meats and brings plenty of the nine essential amino acids but admittedly in poor ratios compared to many other fish.[42]

21. SARDINES (canned) - 1oz = 58.2 cal, **6.9g Protein**, 2%DL SATURATED FAT, 13%DL CHOLESTEROL

Iso	His	Leu	Lys	Met	Phe	Thr	Try	Val
318	203	560	633	278	502	302	77.3	355
4.11	2.62	7.24	8.18	3.59	6.49	3.90	1.00	4.59

Athletes and body builders should take a look at Sardines. They have a good amount of Valine in them and bring surprisingly little Saturated Fat, but they will load you up on Cholesterol, although it is only a third as much as hard-boiled eggs.[62]

22. SCALLOPS (steamed) – 1oz = 31.5 cal, **5.8g Protein**, 0.31%DL SATURATED FAT, 15.5%DL CHOLESTEROL

Iso	His	Leu	Lys	Met	Phe	Thr	Try	Val
195	90	347	357	194	312	177	50	182
3.9	1.8	6.94	7.14	3.89	6.24	3.54	1.00	3.64

Cooked Scallops have higher caloric content because they loose a lot of water during the cooking process compared to the raw ones. Four ounces of steamed scallops will only bring about 1% Daily Limit of Saturated Fat, although they will also bring about 62% DL of Cholesterol, so keep the portions small.[130]

23. SHRIMP (raw, mixed species) – 1oz = 29.7 cal, **5.7g Protein**, 0.42%DL SATURATED FAT, 14%DL CHOLESTEROL

Iso	His	Leu	Lys	Met	Phe	Thr	Try	Val
276	116	451	495	224	429	230	79.2	268
3.48	1.46	5.69	6.25	2.82	5.42	2.90	1.00	3.38

Most sea foods are very low in Saturated Fat and Shrimp are no exception although they will indeed bring plenty of cholesterol. They are low calorie and bring excellent nutrition and a very good array of the nine essential amino acids. The reason for all of the gray and black boxes is their high amount of Tryptophan which skews the rest of the ratios.[132]

24. SPIRULINA (dried) – 1oz = 81.2 cal, **16.1g Protein**, 4%DL SATURATED FAT, 4% FIBER, ZERO CHOLESTEROL

Iso	His	Leu	Lys	Met	Phe	Thr	Try	Val
896	304	1385	847	507	1502	831	260	983
3.44	1.17	5.32	3.25	1.95	5.78	3.19	1.00	3.78

Spirulina is an unusual food bringing Saturated fat and Fiber; quite a rare combination. It comes from the fact that it is blue-green algae also known as cyanobacteria not closely related to either plants or animals and descendants of the first life forms on Earth to develop photosynthesis in order to survive. Spirulina is a true Superfood based on its Vitamin and Mineral content alone. But it is also the densest source of Protein as well bringing about three times as much of the nine essential amino acids per ounce as the second best foods in this list. Vegans can now relax because just 3 ounces of this incredible food will satisfy most of the amino acid requirements of a 200lb adult.[58]

25. SWISS CHEESE (whole milk) – 1oz = 106 cal, **7.5g Protein**, 25%DL SATURATED FAT, 9%DL CHOLESTEROL

Iso	His	Leu	Lys	Met	Phe	Thr	Try	Val
430	298	829	724	301	939	291	112	599
3.83	2.66	7.40	6.46	2.68	8.38+	2.59	1.00	5.34

Unprocessed Swiss Cheese certainly brings a lot of Saturated fat and plenty of Cholesterol, but it is a Superfood when it comes to Calcium and Zinc content. It is also a rich source of very good protein although it is short in Methionine and Threonine.[45]

26. TUNA (light, canned in water) – 1oz = 32.5 cal, **7.1g Protein**, 0.5%DL SATURATED FAT, 3%DL CHOLESTEROL

Iso	His	Leu	Lys	Met	Phe	Thr	Try	Val
329	210	580	656	287	520	313	80.1	368
4.11	2.62	7.24	8.18	3.58	6.49	3.90	1.00	4.59

Tuna is another outstanding fish in terms of nutrient content as well as extremely good ratios of the nine essential amino acids. Add to that the fact that light Tuna canned in water is one of the least expensive meats at your grocery store; this makes Tuna one of the most available, affordable and excellent forms of Complete Protein on the market today.[61]

27. TURKEY (breast, raw) – 1oz = 44 cal, **8.4g Protein**, 1.5%DL SATURATED FAY, 6%DL CHOLESTEROL

Iso	His	Leu	Lys	Met	Phe	Thr	Try	Val
435	261	667	789	329	663	372	95.2	445
4.56	2.74	7.00	8.28	3.46	6.96	3.90	1.00	4.67

While Turkey does have higher amounts of Tryptophan per ounce that many other foods in this list, it is actually in excellent ratios to the rest of the nine essential amino acids. What this means is simply that Turkey has an overall higher density of protein per ounce and a very good concentration of all nine essential amino acids. But it is NOT much higher in Tryptophan than the other foods here and Tryptophan DOES NOT CAUSE DROWSINESS: OVEREATING protein does.[141]

28. YOGURT (whole milk, 8g Protein/cup) – 8 fl. oz. = 149 cal, **8g Protein**, 26%DL SATURATED FAT, 11%DL CHOLESTEROL

Iso	His	Leu	Lys	Met	Phe	Thr	Try	Val
463	211	858	762	328	892	348	49	703
4.6+	2.11	8.58	7.62	3.28	8.92+	3.48	0.5	7.0+

Yogurt is an oddity of the diary products in that it is severely deficient in Tryptophan. The ratios were calculated as if Yogurt has 100mg per cup to prevent the low value from causing all of the others to appear in massive excess. Because of the vast number of different products, protein content and essential amino acid ratios will likely vary greatly.

29. VEAL (shank, lean only, raw) – 1oz = 30.2 cal, **5.4g Protein**, 1%DL SATURATED FAT, 7%DL CHOLESTEROL

Iso	His	Leu	Lys	Met	Phe	Thr	Try	Val
266	196	429	445	187	390	236	54.3	298
4.9+	3.60	7.90	8.19	3.45	7.18+	4.34	1.00	5.48

There is certainly nothing wrong with Veal aside from a couple of the nine essential amino acids in slight excess. In fact, Veal has one of the best Complete Protein profiles in this entire list and comes highly recommended for those who wish to track their amino acids and get them in good proportions.[143]

30. VENISON (loin, lean only, broiled) – 1oz = 42.0 cal, **8.5g Protein**, 1%DL SATURATED FAT, 7%DL CHOLESTEROL

Iso	His	Leu	Lys	Met	Phe	Thr	Try	Val
365	254	647	691	278	587	321	75.3	413
4.8+	3.37	8.59	9.2+	3.69	7.79+	4.26	1.00	5.48

Probably the only knock on lean cuts of Venison is that a few ratios of the essential amino acids are above ideal. Venison is a good source of Choline (31.6mg/oz) and low in Saturated Fat and Cholesterol and is very high in protein density per ounce – only Beef Sirloin, Parmesan Cheese and Spirulina are higher, but all of them have less than ideal ratios – making Deer meat one of the very best sources of Complete Protein.[153]

DOING THE MATH

Example: 180lb Person.

1) Figure out weight in Kilograms: 180 ÷ 2.2 = 81.8kg
2) Daily requirement of Tryptophan: 5mg/kg x 81.8 = 409
3) Find the food you want in the tables above: Example: Turkey. In this table find the essential amino acid with the lowest ratio to Tryptophan (the darkest box) For Turkey this is Leucine.
4) Figure out your daily requirement of Leucine: 409 x 8.6 = 3517mg.
5) Figure out how much Turkey will cover this amount: 3517 ÷ 667mg/oz = 5.27oz. This amount of Turkey (a third of a pound) will cover all of your essential amino acids.
6) Figure out the total amount of Protein, Saturated Fat, Cholesterol and calories this will bring. Assume a 6oz portion of Turkey:
   Protein: 8.4g/oz x 6oz = 50.4g 50g is 100% of the Daily Limit so this is acceptable.
   Sat. Fat: 1.5%DL/oz x 6 = 9% of the Daily Limit. This is excellent.
   Cholesterol: 6%DL/oz x 6 = 36% of the Daily Limit. This should be considered the maximum for those with known

Cholesterol issues. Otherwise it is a very good amount for the day.

Calories: 44cal/oz x 6 = 264 calories. This is a good amount for the daily entrée.

Example: 135lb person.

1) Weight in kilograms: 135lb ÷ 2.2 = 61.3
2) RDA of Tryptophan: 61.3kg x 5mg/kg = 306mg
3) Choose food: Example: Tuna. Leucine is lowest (only gray box.)
4) RDA of Leucine: 306 x 8.6 = 2631mg
5) How much Tuna will cover this? 2631mg ÷ 580mg/oz = 4.5oz
6) Figure out the totals of what this brings (assume whole 5oz can)

Protein: 7.1g/oz x 5 = 35.5g. This is excellent.

Sat. fat: 0.5%DL/oz x 5 = 2.5%DL. This is excellent also.

Cholesterol: 3%DL/oz x 5 = 15%DL. This is excellent as well.

Calories: 32.5cal/oz x 5 = 162.5 calories. This is an excellent amount for the daily entrée.

Example: 150lb Person

1) Weight in kilograms: 150lb ÷ 2.2 = 68.1
2) RDA of Tryptophan: 68.1kg x 5mg/kg = 340mg
3) Choose food: Example: Beef Sirloin. Tryptophan is lowest (dark box)
4) RDA of Tryptophan has already been done: 340mg
5) How much Sirloin will cover this? 340mg ÷ 56.6mg/oz = 6.0oz
6) Figure out the totals of what this brings (assume 6oz steak)

Protein: 8.6g/oz x 6 = 51.6g. This is acceptable.

Sat. fat: 3%DL/oz x 6 = 18%DL. This is good.

Cholesterol: 5%DL/oz x 6 = 30%DL. This is an acceptable maximum amount for those with high cholesterol issues but amounts can VARY.

Calories: 49.6cal/oz x 6 = 297.6 calories. This is a reasonable amount of calories for the daily entrée.

CONCLUSION

Based on our specific needs, fish are the clear winners in terms of bringing the best forms of Complete Protein in the amounts and ratios of the nine essential amino acids to meet our daily dietary requirements. However, it is not necessary to obsess too closely on the exact amounts of the nine essential amino acids in foods that do bring Complete Protein.

For those who do wish to reduce their protein intake, for the purposes of maintaining OPTIMUM THRIVE-LEVEL health; the fish will be of great value because protein is a DIRTY BURNING FUEL that yields very BAD OXIDANTS and no matter how many carbohydrates you eat, the body will always BURN some protein and get about 4 calories per gram out of it. By eating the best forms of Complete Protein (that have the most white boxes) in the least amount needed to get ALL of the nine essential amino acids – you reduce your intake of Saturated Fat, Cholesterol and these bad oxidants in the body.

There are basically six criticisms that I regularly hear concerning the Natural Whole Foods Diet with respect to its nutritional and holistic medicinal benefits. 1) It's too expensive, 2) It's too much trouble to plan, 3) Don't know how to cook, 4) Most of the studies are done on rats and in massive doses that people would never get in a normal diet – study results are not applicable to a "real world" natural whole food diet, and 5) All fresh produce is covered in pesticides which negates the positive health benefits. 6) These healthy foods don't taste as good as the bad foods. Let's look at these concerns one at a time.

"IT'S TOO EXPENSIVE"

This has two problems with it. 1) Not eating right results in illness which is far more expensive and miserable than choosing better food options along the way. 2) The vast majority of the healthy foods in the lists in the preceding chapters are just as cheap as the terrible choices. Cabbage was determined to be the second least expensive fresh vegetable behind only potatoes yet it is a far superior choice as a side dish. Canned Green Beans and Peas can be found in convenience stores and are certainly still two of the least expensive canned goods. Chicken and Turkey breast will certainly be more expensive, but don't sweat the details. If you prefer leg quarters then buy them. They are a bit higher in calories and cholesterol, but roughly the same in nutritional value and a fraction of the cost. Fresh Spinach can be expensive but it doesn't take much to fulfill your daily requirement of Vitamin K. The bottom line here is that you can build a meaningful and healthy diet even on a tight budget by replacing low quality foods with far superior ones that cost nearly the same.

Can't afford the high antioxidant fresh fruits? No problem. Most of my spices come from the local dollar store including Cloves, Oregano, Sage, Cilantro, Paprika, Parsley, Garlic, and Black pepper. All of these have huge ORAC Scores and just a teaspoon of each adds tremendous antioxidant power to anything, even a can of condensed soup – one of the worst products on the shelf of your grocery store: laced with a ton of "un-iodized" salt.

Olive Oil can be a bit expensive too especially now that the science is backing its health promoting power. Add a little to the Canola Oil for a healthier sauté or Oil and Vinegar salad dressing. There's nothing wrong with Canola as salad dressing, it's just stripped of most phytonutrients and nothing but pure calories, but they are in the form of polyunsaturated fats: the good kind.

Shop around a little; it can pay big dividends for your health. I found a good sized bottle of mustard at a discount grocery store that uses Turmeric instead of Yellow #5 making it a powerful medicinal (aside from the sulfur-containing compounds of the Mustard itself) for less than a dollar. The same store has a very inexpensive brand of sour cream which helps me stay away from that awful mayonnaise and its kin.

"IT'S TOO MUCH TROUBLE TO PLAN"

One look at my wife's uncle who didn't know who he was, where he was, or what was in the shampoo bottle he was chugging down, and I realized that I didn't want to spend my last days like that. The modern epidemic diseases cause a lot more trouble than sitting down and figuring out a better and healthier diet that might not cure anything, but it certainly can REDUCE THE RISKS of all of the BIG SEVEN modern epidemic deadly plagues including: Type II diabetes, cardiovascular disease, high cholesterol, high blood pressure, Alzheimer's disease, stroke and cancer. All of these are caused primarily by poor diet over decades of time and when I was in the middle of my poor diet headed towards severe obesity, high blood pressure, high cholesterol and serious blood sugar problems, I KNEW it was a poor diet and I KNEW it was going to kill me. What I did not know back then was that a proper healthy natural whole food diet is easy to plan, inexpensive, and with a little creativity it can be quite delicious too. If you want an easy plan do this: 1) No fast/junk foods, 2) No trash drinks (alcohol or soda), 3) No mayo and its kin, 4) No garbage meats, 5) No high trash calorie sides like potatoes, rice and corn. So you don't have a side dish for dinner any more? Find one. Cabbage is very good: low calorie and high in vitamins C and K, or green beans, green peas, beets, yams, etc. Basically ANYTHING else is better than potatoes, rice and corn.

The reason potatoes, rice and corn comprise 99% of the side dishes in the U.S. is a cultural thing and goes back to when it was a lot harder to shop for food or to be able to afford it, but people do need those 2,000 calories per day in order to function. So these widely available cheap foods loaded with calories became very popular, but they have outlived their usefulness, people just haven't realized this yet. It is no longer the Wild West; there is a major grocery store within a few miles of the vast majority of the people, loaded with far better alternatives at reasonable prices.

"I CAN'T COOK"

Neither could I in the beginning and most of my friends will insist that nothing has changed either. But boiling fresh vegetables like yellow squash is simple. Slice them and toss them in the water and let boil for about 15 minutes. A dash of salt will keep them from being totally bland, but a bigger dash of black pepper and garlic is tasty and much better for you. It is not easy to figure out the amounts of spices to use; but they are too important to ignore. This is certainly not a cookbook but suffice it to say that you do not have to be a nuclear physicist or a gourmet chef to be able to cook quick and simple meals that are both healthy and delicious. But, it will take some time and effort, and if there is a legitimate objection;

this could be it. However, learning to cook for yourself is time and effort very well spent.

"STUDIES ARE NOT REALISTIC"

This is a significant objection mainly because the issue is a bit complicated. Most studies are in their earliest preliminary stages when it comes to testing individual compounds such as Methyl Gallate (has shown very significant anticancer properties.) And even studies on certain foods might be done with mice instead of men, or extracts in test tubes.

. The first issue actually begins with the Big 43 nutrients and the Recommended Daily Allowances published by the Food and Drug Administration. Many of these RDA's were established many decades ago based on the information available at the time. Since then we have made enormous advances in science but that does not necessarily help either because no two studies yield the same results. We know that Vitamin C, the most studied of all human nutritional requirements, is necessary and without it a person will get Scurvy and die. However, the RDA established some time between WWI and WWII (and that has been changed throughout the decades but always staying between 60mg and 95mg/day) is enough to prevent Scurvy, but many researchers believe that this provides BARE MINIMUM SURVIVAL levels of this critical nutrient and nowhere near OPTIMUM THRIVE-LEVEL amounts needed to achieve the best possible health. And the same could be said for any or even all of the Big 43 essential nutrients.

But research has also shown that Vitamin C is water soluble and excesses are routinely eliminated by the kidneys. Therefore taking too much in supplement form will not bring the expected health advantages such as free radical scavenging in the blood stream because the kidneys won't leave it there for long.

Nevertheless, many researchers who have done the studies on Vitamin C insist that the average adult could probably use 500mg as a baseline while recommending anywhere from 1000 to 3000mg. But this is easy to recommend and easy to take as a supplement and difficult to achieve from natural whole foods despite the many foods that bring plenty of it. And some health professionals are calling into question the effectiveness and safety of the synthetic forms of Vitamin C as well indicating that this vitamin has multiple forms and that those found in nature are the ones we need (all plants make the same good forms) while the synthetic ones are a different form (different molecular structures) that might actually be TOXIC. A good amount of fruits daily will bring plenty of Vitamin C (even fruits that are not tart like Bananas and Avocados have some in them) and also brings other powerful antioxidants which have been shown in many studies (possibly the second most studied nutrients in the Big 43) that they can prevent, ameliorate, and even successfully reverse many of the Big Seven modern deadly plagues caused by long term poor diets low in antioxidants.

The argument that mice are not men is fair enough, but they are much more closely related to us than most people would care to know. And in general what is good for them is good for us and what is bad for them is bad for us and vice versa. In fact, they are so closely related to us, deviating by only a few percentage points in their DNA, that they can actually be infected with some human cancer cell lines. Because of this, most tests done on them are testing treatments against HUMAN cancers, not their own. But they have, for example, the same inflammatory markers, signaling pathways, and responses to anti-inflammatory compounds that we do. And this goes for many common maladies including diabetes, high cholesterol, and chemically induced damage to their organs when ameliorated by phytonutrients and the treatments that work for them will almost always have the same positive effects for us as well.

The real issue left is the QUANTITIES of the plants or their extracts that are given to the mice. A study giving them 2000mg per kilogram of body weight will work out to be 160 grams or about 5.6 ounces for a 200lb adult which is a reasonable portion size for many plant foods, but if the mice were given an extract or worse a partial fraction (uses specific solvents to dissolve specific nutrients of the plant, thus concentrating the dosages of those of particular interest) then it is possible that we could never get that much of the specific phytonutrient being studied from natural whole foods.

However, the researchers don't want to conduct their trials for years. These experiments cost money and they need to come to a conclusion within 4 to 8 weeks. Since time is of the essence, they have to use exaggerated doses to see if they can produce any measurable effect in the short time allotted to them. And, by the way, the rats have been given massive doses of the problem that needs to be addressed as well, such as a high-fat diet. In that case they are given nothing but saturated fat to extreme excess as well which no one in their right mind is going to do to themselves and I would argue that in most cases, the two effects cancel each other out anyway. Especially since it is unlikely that the mice are being given an excellent overall diet such that they are getting ALL of the essential nutrients they need in their proper amounts during any study, but we certainly can do that. So by having a far healthier overall diet, the harmful effects that would be caused by say huge quantities of saturated fat and cholesterol are minimized so we don't need concentrated extracts of any plant to help our blood cholesterol levels; just a reasonable portion size with the natural concentrations of the active compounds should do the trick.

So while the study used a huge amount of a given compound and showed positive results, it indicates that as long as we attain and maintain OPTIMUM THRIVE-LEVEL health with a complete

Natural Whole Food Diet, then the limited amounts of the active substances in a natural whole food can and will provide positive and beneficial effects and contribute to that OPTIMUM THRIVE-LEVEL health we seek.

"THE PRODUCE IS COVERED IN PESTICIDES"

I look at the problem of pesticide soaked fresh produce versus packaged foods like this: There is no way to make a blanket statement like: "Pesticides are more poisonous than the additives in packaged foods" or vice versa because EACH chemical has its own specific level of toxicity. In the end, the only way to be fair is to say that both kinds of food contain known proven toxins. If that is to be considered an unavoidable evil of all foods, then the only comparison left is the actual foods themselves. Since packaged and processed foods are for the most part Nonfunctional: have low nutritional or medicinal content and tons of calories, while Natural Whole Foods have much higher nutritional and medicinal content with lower calories (in general and depending on the specific foods) then those are the superior choices. Also, many natural foods like Red Delicious Apples are so loaded with powerful antioxidants that they literally help protect your body from the harmful effects of the pesticide contamination on them while the packaged and processed cookies, chips, and so on have almost no antioxidants in them and expose you to the full damaging effects of their added chemical poisons.

Furthermore and of great significance is the fact that all of the original natural food ingredients in the packaged and processed foods were bathed in pesticides too. So then how well were they washed prior to being processed into the final packaged food product? There is no way to know and the food manufacturers are not obligated to list the pesticides on their product's ingredients on their labels because they didn't add them. In the end, even if they did wash them, the contaminant concentrations will be the same as the fresh produce that you buy and wash for yourself. But the fresh natural whole foods are far more nutritious than any of those packaged, processed and often overcooked food products.

The final deciding factor is that the farmers have no choice but to use those pesticides, otherwise there would be nothing left but dried toothpicks after the locusts finished with their fields. But the packaged and processed food manufacturers DO have a CHOICE and they have chosen to POISON THEIR FOODS. I find that unforgivable and refuse to contribute to their billion dollar bank accounts. Just give it some thought and I think you will agree.

SUPPLEMENT/FOOD PREPARATION

Packaged and processed foods, especially canned goods are notoriously overcooked which in many cases destroys a lot of the nutritional content and antioxidants in the foods. There is no escaping that, but at least they now offer "No Salt Added" versions of the canned products which are important choices because excess Sodium can lead to high blood pressure and it is an FDA regulation that packaged foods cannot use Iodized salt. This was established long ago to keep people from overdosing on Iodine which can be far more serious than chronic shortages.

I am emphasizing natural whole foods and freshly prepared foods rather than supplements because processing foods and dietary supplements has many ways of depleting their nutritional and medicinal value. Cooking definitely depletes vitamin and mineral content but it can also severely deplete antioxidant content as well. This has been demonstrated clearly in the ORAC Scores of many foods that suffer a dramatic decline from the raw score versus the cooked score. Raw Carrots score 697 while Boiled Carrots score 326; a 53% loss of antioxidant power. But, every rule has its exceptions. Boiled Cabbage is higher: 856, than Raw: 529 and at least one source mentions that Lycopene in Tomatoes becomes stronger when they are cooked noting that the Lycopene molecules become "bent" and more potent antioxidants because of this. The ORAC Scores are 423 for cooked "Red Ripe variety" and 387 for the same variety raw; support the claim. Most varieties of fresh apples with skin score between 2,589 and 4,275, but the only entry for a cooked apple product is for apple pie which scored 190 demonstrating a severe depletion regardless of how much crust was included in the test.

Another problem which is specific to antioxidants is exposure to air during processing. While some antioxidants will not suffer much depletion from exposure to the air, others can be severely depleted. Apple sauce scored 1,965 which was better than expected, but it does show a decline due to processing and turning brown versus eating fresh white pulp apples with their skin. Apple Juice (again just one entry in the source list so the brand name and preparation techniques are unknown) scored just 414 and may indicate severe loss of antioxidant potential due to the further processing and possibly heating involved in its production. Since all varieties of apples lose over 20% of their scores when peeled, this is a possible cause of the reduction in antioxidant power in apple sauce (which has lost even more than that) while apple juice is severely low. This indicates that the antioxidants in apples are in higher amounts in and near the skin and could also be relatively insoluble in water so they don't come out into the juice. The severe depletion in antioxidants of the baked apple pie indicates that the prolonged heat of cooking destroys them almost completely.[34]

JUICES, OILS, ETC.

These products are very confusing. Dark grapes (either red or black) have a separate entry for Grape Juice – specifically 100% Concord variety because their nutrient content is different. The juice has an ORAC score of 2,389 while black grapes (no specific variety information mentioned) score 1,746.[34] Welch's brand labeling on the bottle indicates that they use 550 grapes in the 64 oz bottle amounting to about 68 grapes per 8oz serving. Since an 8oz serving brings 32% Chromium, and 1 cup of whole grapes is about 20 of them, a little math yields 1.16%DV of Chromium per cup of fresh grapes. This makes the juice a far better choice not only for Chromium but also for its higher antioxidant power as well. However, all reliable sources also indicate that the skins are the exclusive source of many of the grapes powerful active ingredients like Resveratrol. This puts the dark grapes, and dark raisins, back in contention and you should try to include them in your diet now and then as well.

Cranberries score very high: 9,090, but the unsweetened juice only scores 1,452 which indicates another fruit with antioxidants concentrated in the skins or that are relatively insoluble in water and don't come out of the solids when the fruits are squeezed, just like apples.[34] This does not diminish the benefits of Cranberry juice; that score is still excellent and its health promoting unique phytonutrients are present in the juice. But the practical upshot is that eating fresh whole fruits is sometimes better and different from the juices, but the juices are still infinitely superior to drinking crud like soda pop.

Just about all vegetable oils on the shelf of your grocery store are refined. The refining process heats the oil and also purposely removes as many of the plants original phytonutrients as possible in order to render a more "neutral" or tasteless and odorless oil. In many cases this is preferable in cooking. For example, frying eggs, which are rather bland flavored, would be overwhelmed by the taste of most raw and unrefined oils.

However, because most of the plant's original phytonutrients have been removed, whatever health benefits the oil could have brought have been lost as well. This applies to Olive oil, Sesame seed oil and Coconut oil in particular but all oils lose phytonutrients in the refining process. Neutral, odorless or refined Coconut oil might as well be corn oil (total crud by the way, so try to switch to Canola, it is a far healthier much lighter refined oil.) If you can't find "Cold expeller" pressed Coconut Oil at your local grocery store then search for it online; there are many vendors who will gladly ship it to you and it is worth the cost and the effort. The same holds for Sesame Seed Oil although the Sesame Seed Butter, called Tahini, is the far better choice for being able to incorporate it into your diet (i.e. a delightful spread for whole grain toast.)

Finally, dried fruit, even Apples score as much as 45% higher in antioxidant power than the plain fresh fruits. This is a boon that puts these excellent snack choices into serious contention as some of the better ways to get in on these fruits powerful health benefits. Four of the very best choices are: Dried Plums (Prunes,) Dried Apricots, Raisins and "Craisins" (dried Cranberries) that provide you with a convenient way to add the health promoting powers of these excellent fruits to your regular diet.

Extracts and partial extracts called fractions are yet another source of confusion. Some extracts may be excellent and superior forms of the natural plant. In fact, there are many medicinal herbs that should only be taken as extracts in supplement form for many reasons including: too strong to mess with raw, too variable (some plants vary dramatically in their active compounds concentrations even between two plants grown side by side,) or the raw plant is actually toxic until properly processed. Two good examples of plants that are too toxic in their raw forms are Olives which must be cured and Agave which must be processed into a honey-like sweetener which is what gets fermented into Tequila. But it has become a popular alternative sweetener even though it still has a high Glycemic Index.

However, many extracts are coming up short of the mark. I know my Gingko biloba supplements from just five years ago were substantially more effective than the one I am taking now that claims to be "4:1 Standardized Extract." These standardized extracts are being produced by wholesalers that sell them to the supplement manufacturers who simply load them into the capsules and count them into the bottles, stick on the labels and ship them out to retailers. Having the actual preparation of the extracts done by another company might save a lot of time and money, but it is also a mystery as to what was done to the product in its creation. This is clearly a problem of "too many cooks in the kitchen" which wrecks the pills.

Many products are being offered as fractions now which are simply extracts done with specific solvents like ethylene, which tend to pull or dissolve only some specific molecules out of the pulverized plant matter rather than everything. The idea is that the fraction will result in a much higher concentration of the desired phytonutrients but I have found that while this works in the original scientific studies, the retail products are often very weak because they are not using nearly enough of the original plant matter to produce the expected concentrations so they are not as effective as the substances used in the studies and bring more grandiose claims than they do results. Also, many phytonutrients turn out to be far more effective in their freshest possible forms that are most complete and often lose their effectiveness when certain "active" compounds are isolated. This has been noted from time to time in studies as a possible "synergistic effect." This simply means that it is the combination of the various substances in the original plant that work together to produce the desired effect. In fact, Traditional Chinese Medicine is based on this synergism which is why over the centuries the practitioners have tested various combinations of their ingredients in order to maximize this effect and make their formulas stronger and more effective. Sometimes these isolated active compounds can actually turn detrimental as well such as

Aspirin which will knock holes in your stomach while Willow bark tea (the original natural source) is not as harsh.

THE SUPPLEMENT MARKET

The key is not to get dazzled by the hype and run out and spend an obscene amount of money on some purported miracle cure. Dietary supplements right now are basically the Wild West. There is very little regulation on them. The most the FDA does is to test them to be sure they do not contain any patented, controlled or banned substances or exceed the established limits of known toxins and contaminants (you don't want to know the amount of "insect parts, eggs, larvae, etc." that is permitted.) Second, they make sure that the product makes no claims that the agency has not already validated as legitimate. And finally, they make certain that no one ever claims to be able to cure cancer: do that and you go straight to jail. After that the manufacturers can pretty much do what they want. This is exactly why there are literally hundreds of manufacturers that I have tracked down resulting in about TEN THOUSAND product types like Vitamin A pills, Vitamin B1 pills, etc. And some of these types of products are offered by many hundreds of different companies resulting in possibly a HUNDRED THOUSAND or more individual dietary supplement products on the market today.

This is not to say that they don't work. Most small companies are started by good people who have learned something and decided to make it into a product so that everyone can get in on the benefits of their discovery. But, there are simply not enough hours in the day to be able to take one of each TYPE of dietary supplement out there and quite frankly I believe that many of them are for the most part unnecessary. But not because the product doesn't provide anything; almost all of them do provide something of value. I believe most products are unnecessary because natural whole foods are more than sufficient to meet our needs of almost everything. And they will bring those things in superior forms and amounts while supplements often contain synthetics of dubious bioavailability and safety and are much more likely to be taken in excess which is by far the leading cause of adverse reactions and poisoning caused by something that should improve the person's health, not wreck it.

There are specific cases when the supplement is the best way to go. If you want MORE Omega-3 DHA and EPA than what one teaspoon of Cod Liver Oil will provide (888mg which is very good and cost effective when compared to the cost of a Vitamin A pill, and a Vitamin D3 pill and a DHA/EPA pill) then you should add the supplement pills rather than take additional quantities of the Cod Liver Oil which is very high in Vitamin A as Retinol and overdosing on this form can lead to adverse toxic reactions which are not pleasant to say the least and certainly not worth suffering through when the goal is to improve your health, not ruin it.

The same can be said for virtually all of the minerals. These are almost all metals and in supplement form they are almost all synthetic, even the chelates. And these synthetics should never be taken in amounts above 100% RDA daily. All of these metals can become TOXIC in excess, not just Copper. Even if I was living on nothing but instant noodles, I would skip a day between taking any mineral supplement even if they were just 100% RDA amounts mainly to be on the safe side. But you must also remember that many whole foods bring a lot more vitamins and minerals than what I have listed, but less than 10% which I did not include in my listings because they are not significant quantities for the purposes of building a natural whole food diet plan for the day aiming at getting all of the Big 43 in 100% RDA amounts. I did keep the amounts for Fiber (and Chromium) even below 10% because it is difficult to get in the 100% RDA amount of Fiber daily if you do not include Black Beans, Lentils or Mung Beans on that day.

Some supplements do bring very measurable and significant health benefits and medicinal properties in very convenient forms rather than messing around with whole plants or preparing herbal teas from dried bulk products and are worth considering. Artichoke Leaf extract contains the Caffeoylquinic acid and has been shown to be a very effective liver detoxification agent and comes highly recommended mainly because this active compound is mainly in the leaves and not the normally available edible part of the plant.

Many plants that are available have this quality; another part of the plant not normally available or eaten, has been found in studies to provide significant health benefits. And for those who do not wish to try to make herbal teas, the supplements are the best alternative although 100% pure dried bulk herb, when available is far better and quite often less expensive.

BEST PRACTICES

1. HAVE A PLAN – The plan is to transform your daily dietary regimen for the rest of your life, You do not want to "go on a diet" in order to suffer through it to finally reach your target level of health, then relax and end up where you started.

2. REPLACE THE BAD WITH THE GOOD – Start with snacks. I snack often and by replacing chips and dip, cookies, etc. with low calorie alternatives like celery, carrots and even pickles this resulted in an immediate and drastic reduction in daily caloric intake (by several THOUSAND calories per day) as well as a huge improvement in overall health by adding the antioxidant power of the carrots and the medicinal power of the celery.

3. TRANSFORM ONE MEAL AT A TIME – Breakfast is the easiest one to change. It should be oatmeal and add a few table spoons of Wheat Germ now and then. Add sliced fresh fruits and sweeten with raw bee honey or Stevia (the packets are terrible, but it doesn't take much fresh leaf Stevia to make the bowl sweet.) Lunch is also easy: it should be a tossed salad adorned with Oil and Vinegar dressing. For dinner replace the potatoes, rice, and corn and other nonfunctional side dishes with an assortment of the Net Negative Calorie foods, Even 8 ounces of many different kinds of fish will still bring far fewer calories than most other land animal meats and they are far better for you because they all bring some of the Omega-3 Fatty Acids DHA and EPA.

4. HUNT FOR BETTER CHOICES – It is an ongoing process. Always be on the lookout for better supplements, spices (that are powerhouses of antioxidants and medicinal phytonutrients) and fresh fruits and vegetables (also usually low calorie with high nutritional and medicinal value.) Many folks get "stuck in a flavor rut" and don't like to try new foods. I was like that but now I am the opposite; I am eager to try new foods and many turn out to be exquisite. I have run into my share of foods I don't like very much as well, but that is what garlic, onions, bell peppers and the spices were invented for: to repair a food's flavor and if that doesn't work, then they can overwhelm it.

5. DON'T SWEAT THE DETAILS – If you stick to the plan and replace high calorie foods with low calorie foods and low nutritional value foods with high nutritional value foods – dump nonfunctional foods for the Functional foods – then you will definitely experience a tangible improvement in your overall health. Having boiled spinach and green peas as sides for dinner, you know they don't add up to a lot of calories, so a second helping of both will not take you way over the top: and that is the key to sticking with the Net Negative Calorie foods. They make staying fit and healthy easy and fun because you don't have to always run to the nutrition label and calculate how many calories are in the serving you want to eat. When it comes to cucumbers, you can eat them until you turn green, and still probably haven't passed a few dozen calories worth. And when transforming your every day eating lifestyle in this way you don't have to worry about your health any more. Trust the Natural Whole Foods Diet foods to do their jobs and they will deliver the desired results.

LAST THOUGHTS

The main objections to the natural Whole Foods Diet are: 1) It's too expensive, 2) It takes too much time, 3) Don't know-how to cook, 4) Grocery store produce is covered in pesticides which is at least as toxic as packaged foods.

I have known many people who eat very well – proper Natural Whole Food diets – on Food Stamps. I am not suggesting a diet of Live Maine Lobster and Filet Mignon every night; I am suggesting simply to pay closer attention to the amounts of Nonfunctional foods loaded with trash calories and little nutritional or medicinal value in your diet and replace the bad foods with good ones. A can of No Salt added Green Peas rather than Pinto beans literally costs no extra and as you go through your diet making these replacements in every meal, they add up to a far superior regular dietary regimen that can literally save your life.

As for cooking skill, I assure you that I started out incapable of boiling water or frying an egg. Even now I would not call myself a "Chef" but it doesn't take much skill or time (about 15 minutes) to boil a pot of sliced yellow squash (a great Net Negative Calorie Food) either. It does take time to learn to cook things and I wasted half a bag of dried Lentils before I got the hang of cooking them, but it was well worth the effort: they have an ORAC score of over 7,000 making them TEN TIMES stronger in antioxidant power than raw carrots.[34] The key is not to jump into the deep end of the pool with cook books featuring dishes like Chocolate Mousse (one of the most difficult dishes to get right) but instead just keep things simple like the boiled yellow squash. As you progress you can learn how to make your favorite dishes along the way.

It is very tempting and very easy to overdose on the essential nutrients when taken in supplement form: DO NOT OVERDOSE on them because MORE IS NEVER BETTER when it comes to STRONG MEDICINE and the essential nutrients are indeed strong medicine for the human body. You can go higher than the RDA amounts of the following: ANTIOXIDANTS (in foods ONLY, NOT supplements,) VITAMIN A (but ONLY BETA-CAROTENE and other Carotenoids and ONLY from plant foods,) VITAMIN C (preferably from foods and not supplements,) OMEGA-3 FATTY ACIDS (the ONLY essential nutrients that I recommend in large doses from supplements,) and all of the B VITAMINS try to get as much as you can from natural whole foods and do not go beyond 200% from NATURAL EXTRACT SOURCE supplements.) The rest should all be kept at no more than 100% RDA amounts on a long-term daily basis including ALL MINERALS, VITAMIN A (as RETINOL,) VITAMIN D3, VITAMIN E, and VITAMIN K.

Pay close attention to Saturated Fat and Cholesterol. While Cholesterol comes exclusively from animal products, many plants (mostly seeds, nuts and oils) bring Saturated Fats as well as the unsaturated fats. And keeping these two from getting out of hand will result in excellent long-term health benefits by reducing high blood pressure, high cholesterol, and the risk of cardiovascular disease.

Try to reduce the portions of foods that have high Glycemic Index values. For those that did not have the GI value data, watch the CL – Carb Load. Foods with a CL of less than 10% are good, and a CL of less than 3% is outstanding; such foods will not mess with your blood sugar regulatory and metabolism systems and help you to avoid Type II Diabetes.

As you read through the lists of foods including: 84 natural whole foods and spices and their ORAC scores, 121 Functional Foods and their nutrient and phytonutrient content, it should have become clear that almost every single time a phytonutrient was mentioned it invariably brought the ability to reduce the risk of or ameliorate the symptoms of at least one but usually several of the BIG SEVEN modern deadly epidemic plagues: high cholesterol, high blood pressure, cardiovascular disease, Alzheimer's disease, Type II Diabetes, Stroke (cerebrovascular disease, is the fancy name and it includes aneurisms as well) and Cancer.

It literally takes a lot of work to AVOID the hundreds of foods that can help you to avoid these terrible afflictions! The problem is the dietary cultural RUT of eating nothing but POTATOES, RICE and CORN as side dishes for everything. I am not saying that they are devoid of nutritional value, what I am saying is that these three are eaten almost to the complete EXCLUSION of anything and everything else; and that is a problem because all preparations of these three menaces have dangerously high Glycemic index values – they are the BIG THREE FOOD CAUSES OF TYPE II DIABETES. And because everyone is eating just them and none of the other foods in the 121 Functional Foods List, then they are not getting any of the foods that can help reduce the risks of the BIG SEVEN plagues and that's why those diseases – RARE 70 years ago – have EXPLODED into EPIDEMICS today.

Heart disease (and heart failure as a result of it) killed over 650,000 people in the U.S. in 2016. It is the #1 Cause of Death in the U.S. now and it is NOT a death by natural cause; it is death due to decades of MALNUTRITION – oh, we eat a LOT of food and a LOT of CALORIES, but all of that food contains very little NUTRITIONAL value which is why I say "We are the BEST FED, most MALNOURISHED society the world has ever known." We can blame the 598,000 deaths from Cancer in 2016 (the #2 cause of death in the U.S.) on radioactive fallout from three decades of nuclear bomb testing followed by the Chernobyl and Fukushima reactor accidents, but all of that pollution has NOTHING TO DO WITH cardiovascular disease – that's on US and our HORRIFIC eating habits. A TRASH DIET leads to TRASHED HEALTH and an EARLY GRAVE. High blood pressure which places a terrible strain on the Heart, which never gets a break or a day off, will KILL YOU. High cholesterol in the blood leads to Atherosclerosis, plaque build up on the blood vessel walls that constricts them and raises blood pressure, increasng the strain on the heart, and it will KILL YOU. And there are no nasty little viruses doing this and there is no "Atherosclerosis gene" to blame: it is horrible diet over decades of time. If the BIG SEVEN are due to poor diet and killing 1,571,000 people per year, and it takes at least 30 years for poor diet to take a person from good health to life-threatening symptoms, then right now over 47 MILLION people are standing in that line… eating their way to death. You do not have to be a part of that any more.

THANK YOU AND GOD BLESS AND GOOD LUCK AND ABOVE ALL ELSE: TAKE CARE OF YOURSELF! (BECAUSE NO ONE ELSE IS GOING TO DO IT)

ANNIE'S REMEDY

WEBSITE: www.anniesremedy.com

A valuable online source of information with well over 300 plants listed in their database which was instrumental in the writing of this book. They also sell high quality Essential Oils.

Dr. Godofredo Stuart, Jr. M.D.

WEBSITE: www.stuartxchange.org

This is one of the largest databases of medicinal plants (800+ plants) on the Internet and a valuable tool without which I would not have been able to write this book.

THE FDA and the NIH

U.S. Food and Drug Administration: www.fda.gov

National Institutes for Health: www.nih.gov

Both of these governmental agencies have informative websites. Like all governmental agencies, their websites can be difficult to navigate and much of the material is either too simplified or too complicated to be of much value, but I still recommend that you visit them and take a look around.

Dr. James Duke's Phytochemical & Ethnobotanical Database

WEBSITE: https://phytochem.nal.usda.gov/phytochem/search/list

Kept at the USDA's website, this has the detailed chemical analysis of over 2,000 plants.

"DR. AXE"

WEBSITE: www.draxe.com

Josh Axe has an extensive website which I have used as a primary base source of most of the information on the essential nutrients, whole foods health benefits, and unbiased reports on many supplements, that includes excellent explanations of what each nutrient is, the health benefits of each one, the nasty results of chronic deficiency for each one, and a list of foods that contain them. The website covers a lot of ground too, not just the "ABC's" (the vitamins and minerals) but also many other health food items and supplements like Lycopene, Milk Thistle, and fad products like Creatine, etc. This website comes highly recommended.

"MY FOOD DATA"

WEBSITE: www.myfooddata.com

This is another superb website although they don't get too deep into the nature of each nutrient and it is far from complete like "Dr. Axe" but they do have excellent lists of the top foods that contain each essential nutrient that they do cover and it is a good source of that specific information and I highly recommend that you check it out too.

THE GEORGE MATELJAN FOUNDATION

WEBSITE: www.whfoods.org

This is one of the best reference websites that covers many minerals in excellent detail that most other websites do not. They include a lot of good information on the function of most of the nutrients in the body as well, some of which I could only find at this website and I could never have written this book without their vast collection of nutritional information. They include a lot of additional and useful information about the individual natural whole foods including recipes and weekly diet plans. Check it out.

WIKIPEDIA
WEBSITE: www.wikipedia.org

Often maligned because "anybody" can start an entry or edit an existing entry, Wikipedia is by far the largest repository of general information on every conceivable subject on planet Earth. It is an enormous encyclopedia and while some entries on the subject of nutrients are rather limited and also include a lot of talk about the molecular structures and chemistry like methods of synthesis and so on, it is still one of the best online resources that covers all subjects and each page does include the references which you can pursue as well. Whenever they ask for a few dollars, please give, so we can keep this vast repository of information free and unencumbered by advertising.

"SUPERFOODLY"
WEBSITE ADDRESS: www.superfoodly.com

This site lists the ORAC – Oxygen Radical Absorption Capacity – scores for hundreds of different foods, mostly natural whole foods. While the ORAC score was invented to measure the antioxidant potential of foods compared to each other side-by-side (the ORAC score is based on 100 grams of each food) it is not absolute because not all antioxidants are the same. The thing to remember is not to use the information to replace one food item with another, but to add powerful antioxidant-rich foods to your regular eating regimen. For example, Cloves have one of the highest scores of all commonly available food items, 290,283, while carrots have an ORAC score of 697. But you can't replace a medium sized carrot with a gram of cloves because the carrots bring beta-Carotene which for many people is the only way they are going to get their daily requirement of Vitamin A. I highly recommend this website as a way to "shop for" new antioxidant-rich foods to add to your natural whole foods diet.

NUTRITION DATA at SELF.COM
WEBSITE: http://nutritiondata.self.com

I am not sure if I could even write this book without this website. They have one of the largest repositories of detailed nutrient analyses of a wide range of foods, both packaged as well as natural whole foods, imaginable. The original source of the data is the FDA website, but this website has it in a far better format. You can search for many natural whole foods and they will most likely have the complete nutrition label including every vitamin, mineral, and many other nutrients as well as "undesirable" constituents listed in that label including cholesterol and saturated fat.

Unfortunately, those labels do lack Molybdenum and Iodine (both covered at the George Mateljan Foundation's website) but the total information provided for each food is still very useful. I have this one bookmarked so I can quickly check the nutritional value of any food at any time.

"WEB MD"

WEBSITE ADDRESS: www.webmd.com

Aside from having an extensive collection of articles on the nutrients, WebMD also includes many articles on prevention and treatment for just about every ailment as well. I couldn't remember where I had heard that turkey causes drowsiness on Thanksgiving because of its high levels of LACTIC ACID and overindulgence of it at the Thanksgiving dinner table and that it is NOT caused by Tryptophan. In a general Google search, WebMD was near the top of the list with an article that confirmed that Tryptophan – an ESSENTIAL AMINO ACID found in ALL PROTEINS in ALL CELLS in YOUR BODY and with higher concentrations in Chicken than Turkey – is NOT the cause of drowsiness EVER: OVEREATING Complete Protein (animal source protein) is the cause they lay out and I still can't find where I read that it was the lactic acid! But the point is that WebMD is a great source of health related information and I definitely have it bookmarked on all of my computers.

SOURCES OF DIETARY/HERBAL SUPPLEMENTS

I have not been able to check most of the manufacturers out because there are literally many hundreds of them. You will have to verify the quality and authenticity of their products by searching for neutral third party reviews of their products (such as Consumer Reports.)

VITACOST – www.vitacost.com – This is a large online dietary supplement and natural foods vendor. They carry hundreds of brands and manufacture some high quality products of their own.

NOW FOODS – www.nowfoods.com – An excellent high quality dietary supplement manufacturer.

JARROW FORMULAS – www.jarrow.com – This is another manufacturer of very high quality dietary supplements.

SWANSON VITAMINS – www.swansonvitamins.com – While they do carry many other brands, this company makes a lot of holistic herbal supplements, many of which can't be found anywhere else.

GARDEN of LIFE – www.gardenoflife.com – This company makes a whole line of supplements based on natural extract sources of very high quality; many of their products have no competition that I could find: no other natural extract product of the same nutrient(s) on the market, just synthetics. Some of their products are never exposed to temperatures above 115°F which would destroy many nutrients during manufacture. The products are not inexpensive but they are definitely the very best that I could find.

REFERENCES

[1] The data on Vitamin A was found at: * https://draxe.com/top-10-vitamin-foods/ Retrieved 7/23/18 * https://www.myfooddata.com/articles/food-sources-of-vitamin-A.php Retrieved 7/23/18 * www.whfoods.com /genpage.php?tname=nutrient&dbid=106 Retrieved 7/23/18

[2] Vitamin B1 - Thiamine: https://draxe.com/thiamine-foods/ Retrieved 7/23/18 * https://ods.od.nih.gov/factsheets/Thiamin-HealthProfessional/ Retrieved 7/23/18

[3] Vitamin B2 – Riboflavin: https://draxe.com/vitamin-b2/ Retrieved 7/23/18 * https://www.myfooddata.com/articles/foods-high-in-riboflavin-vitamin-B2.php Retrieved 7/23/18 * http://www.whfoods.com /genpage.php?tname=nutrient&dbid=93 Retrieved 7/23/18 * https://ods.od.nih.gov/factsheets/Riboflavin-HealthProfessional/ Retrieved 7/23/18

[4] Vitamin B3 - Niacin: https://draxe.com/niacin-side-effects/ Retrieved 7/24/18 * https://www.myfooddata.com/articles/foods-high-in-niacin-vitamin-B3.php Retrieved 7/24/18 * http://www.whfoods.com /genpage.php?tname=nutrient&dbid=83 Retrieved 7/24/18

[5] Vitamin B5 – Pantothenic acid: https://draxe.com/vitamin-b5/ Retrieved 7/24/18 * http://www.whfoods.com/genpage.php?tname=nutrient &dbid=87 Retrieved 7/24/18 * https://en.wikipedia.org/wiki/ Pantothenic_acid Retrieved 7/24/18

[6] Vitamin B6 - Pyridoxine: https://draxe.com/top-10-vitamin-b6-foods/ Retrieved 7/24/18 * http://www.whfoods.com/genpage.php?tname= nutrient&dbid=108 Retrieved 7/24/18

[7] Vitamin B7 - Biotin: https://draxe.com/biotin-benefits/ Retrieved 7/24/18 * https://en.wikipedia.org/wiki/Biotin Retrieved 7/24/18 * http://www.whfoods.com/genpage.php?tname=nutrient&dbid=42

[8] Vitamin B9 - Folic acid: * https://draxe.com/top-10-vitamin-b9-folate-foods/ Retrieved 7/24/18 * http://www.whfoods.com/genpage.php? tname=nutrient&dbid=63 Retrieved 7/24/18

[9] Vitamin B12 - Methylcobalamin: * https://draxe.com/vitamin-b12-benefits/ Retrieved 7/24/18 * https://en.wikipedia.org/wiki/Cobalamin Retrieved 7/24/18

[10] Choline: * https://draxe.com/what-is-choline/ Retrieved 7/24/18 * http://www.whfoods.com/genpage.php?tname=nutrient&dbid=50 Retrieved 7/24/18

[11] Vitamin C – l-Ascorbic acid: * https://draxe.com/vitamin-c-benefits/ Retrieved 7/26/18 * https://www.myfooddata.com/articles/vitamin-c-foods.php Retrieved 7/26/18 * http://www.whfoods.com/genpage.php? tname=nutrient&dbid=109 Retrieved 7/26/18

[12] Vitamin D3 – Cholecalciferol: https://draxe.com/vitamin-d-deficiency-symptoms/ Retrieved 7/26/18 * https://www.myfooddata.com/articles /high-vitamin-D-foods.php Retrieved 7/26/18 * www.whfoods.com /genpage.php?tname=nutrient&dbid=110 Retrieved 7/26/18

[13] Vitamin E – alpha-Tocopherol: https://draxe.com/vitamin-e-foods/ Retrieved 7/26/18 * https://www.myfooddata.com/articles/vitamin-e-foods.php Retrieved 7/26/18 * http://www.whfoods.com/genpage.php ?tname=nutrient&dbid=111 Retrieved 7/26/18

[14] Vitamin K – n-Quinones: * https://draxe.com/vitamin-k-deficiency/ Retrieved 7/26/18 * https://www.myfooddata.com/articles/food-sources-of-vitamin-k.php Retrieved 7/26/18 * www.whfoods.com/ genpage.php?tname=nutrient&dbid=112 Retrieved 7/26/18

[15] Calcium: https://draxe.com/foods-high-in-calcium/ Retrieved 7/30/18 *
https://www.myfooddata.com/articles/foods-high-in-calcium.php
Retrieved 7/30/18 * http://www.whfoods.com/genpage.php?tname
=nutrient&dbid=45 Retrieved 7/30/18

[16] Fiona S. Atkinson, Kaye Foster-Powell, and Jennie C. Brand-Miller,
"International tables of glycemic index and glycemic load values:
2008": Diabetes Care, Vol. 31, number 12, pg 2281-2283, American
Diabetes Association © Dec. 2008.

[17] Chromium: * https://draxe.com/what-is-chromium/ Retrieved 8/23/18 *
http://www.whfoods.com/genpage.php?tname=nutrient&dbid=51
Retrieved 8/23/18

[18] Copper: * https://draxe.com/foods-high-in-copper/ Retrieved 8/23/18 *
https://www.myfooddata.com/articles/high-copper-foods.php
Retrieved 8/23/18 * http://www.whfoods.com/genpage.php?tname
=nutrient&dbid=53 Retrieved 8/23/18

[19] Iodine: * https://draxe.com/iodine-rich-foods/ Retrieved 7/26/18 *
https://www.myfooddata.com/articles/natural-foods-high-in-iodine.php
Retrieved 7/26/18

[20] Iron: * https://draxe.com/top-10-iron-rich-foods/ Retrieved 7/30/18 *
https://www.myfooddata.com/articles/food-sources-of-iron.php
Retrieved 7/30/18 * http://www.whfoods.com/genpage.php?tname
=nutrient&dbid=70 Retrieved 7/30/18

[21] Magnesium: * https://draxe.com/magnesium-deficient-top-10-
magnesium-rich-foods-must-eating/ Retrieved 7/30/18 *
https://www.myfooddata.com/articles/foods-high-in-magnesium.php
Retrieved 7/30/18 * http://www.whfoods.com/genpage.php?tname
=nutrient&dbid=75 Retrieved 7/30/18

[22] Manganese: * https://draxe.com/manganese/ Retrieved 8/23/18 *
https://www.myfooddata.com/articles/foods-high-in-manganese.php
Retrieved 8/23/18

[23] Molybdenum: * http://www.whfoods.com/genpage.php?tname=
nutrient&dbid=128 Retrieved 8/29/18

[24] Phosphorus: * https://draxe.com/foods-high-in-phosphorus/ Retrieved
7/30/18 * https://www.myfooddata.com/articles/high-phosphorus-
foods.php Retrieved 7/30/18 * http://www.whfoods.com/genpage.php?
tname=nutrient&dbid=127 Retrieved 7/30/18

[25] Potassium: * https://draxe.com/low-potassium/ Retrieved 8/23/18 *
https://www.myfooddata.com/articles/food-sources-of-potassium.php
Retrieved 8/23/18

[26] Selenium: * https://draxe.com/selenium-foods/ Retrieved 8/23/18 *
https://www.myfooddata.com/articles/foods-high-in-selenium.php
Retrieved 8/23/18 * http://www.whfoods.com/genpage.php?tname
=nutrient&dbid=95 Retrieved 8/23/18

[27] Sodium: * https://draxe.com/low-potassium/ Retrieved 8/23/18

[28] Sulfur: https://articles.mercola.com/sites/articles/archive/2016/05/16/
sulfur-in-the-body.aspx Retreived on 01-03-2019

[29] Zinc: * https://draxe.com/foods-high-in-zinc/ Retrieved 8/23/18 *
https://www.myfooddata.com/articles/high-zinc-foods.php Retrieved
8/23/18 * http://www.whfoods.com/genpage.php?tname=nutrient
&dbid=115 Retrieved 8/23/18

[30] Walnuts: https://nutritiondata.self.com/facts/nut-and-seed-
products/3138/2 Retrieved 9/12/18

[31] Almonds: https://nutritiondata.self.com/facts/nut-and-seed-
products/3087/2 Retrieved 9/12/18

[32] Sunflower seed kernels: https://nutritiondata.self.com/facts/nut-and-seed-products/3077/2 Retrieved 9/12/18

[33] Peanuts and peanut butter: https://nutritiondata.self.com/facts/legumes-and-legume-products/4453/2 Retrieved 9/12/18

[34] Antioxidants: https://draxe.com/top-10-high-antioxidant-foods/ Retrieved 8/20/18 * http://www.superfoodly.com (ORAC scores) Retrieved 8/29/18

[35] Kiwi: https://nutritiondata.self.com/facts/fruits-and-fruit-juices/1934/2 Retrieved 9/12/18

[36] Grapefruit: https://nutritiondata.self.com/facts/fruits-and-fruit-juices/1905/2 Retrieved 9/12/18 * www.anniesremedy.com/citrus-paradisi-grapefruit.php Retrieved 12/20/18 * www.stuartxchange.org/Suha.html Retrieved 12/5/18

[37] Cabbage: https://nutritiondata.self.com/facts/vegetables-and-vegetable-products/2372/2 Retrieved 9/12/18 * www.stuartxchange.org/Repolyo.html Retrieved 12/5/18

[38] Carrots: https://nutritiondata.self.com/facts/vegetables-and-vegetable-products/2383/2 Retrieved 9/12/18 * www.stuartxchange.org/Karot.html

[39] Black Beans: https://nutritiondata.self.com/facts/legumes-and-legume-products/4287/2 Retrieved 3/8/19 * http://whfoods.com/genpage.php?tname=foodspice&dbid=2 Retrieved 3/8/19

[40] Blackeye Peas: https://nutritiondata.self.com/facts/legumes-and-legume-products/4333/2 Retrieved 3/8/19

[41] Blueberry: http://whfoods.com/genpage.php?tname=foodspice&dbid=8 Retrieved 3/8/19 * https://draxe.com/pterostilbene/ Retrieved 3/8/19

[42] Salmon: https://nutritiondata.self.com/facts/ethnic-foods/10460/2 Retrieved 9/12/18

[43] Wheat germ: https://nutritiondata.self.com/facts/cereal-grains-and-pasta/5743/2 Retrieved 9/12/18

[44] Parmesan (and Romano) cheese: https://nutritiondata.self.com/facts/dairy-and-egg-products/32/2 Retrieved 9/12/18

[45] Swiss cheese: https://nutritiondata.self.com/facts/dairy-and-egg-products/39/2 Retrieved 9/12/18

[46] Yogurt: https://nutritiondata.self.com/facts/dairy-and-egg-products/104/2 Retrieved 9/12/18

[47] Cod Liver Oil: https://nutritiondata.self.com/facts/fats-and-oils/628/2 Retrieved 9/12/18

[48] Beef liver: https://nutritiondata.self.com/facts/beef-products/3468/2 Retrieved 9/12/18

[49] Broccoli: https://nutritiondata.self.com/facts/vegetables-and-vegetable-products/2356/2 Retrieved 9/12/18

[50] Grapes, grape seed, and grape juice: https://draxe.com/grapes-nutrition/ Retrieved 9/12/18 * www.anniesremedy.com/vitis-vinifera-grapes.php Retrieved 12/20/18 * https://nutritiondata.self.com/facts/fruits-and-fruit-juices/1923/2

[51] Garlic: https://www.webmd.com/vitamins/ai/ingredientmono-300/garlic Retrieved 9/18/18 * www.anniesremedy.com/allium-sativum-garlic.php Retrieved 12/20/18 * www.stuartxchange.org/Bawang.html Retrieved 12/5/18

[52] The 9 Essential Amino Acids: * https://bareblends.com.au/blog/the-9-essential-amino-acids-what-are-they-and-why-do-we-need-them/ Retrieved 8/23/18 * http://en.wikipedia.org/Essential_amino_acid Retrieved 3/26/19

[53] Oysters: https://nutritiondata.self.com/facts/finfish-and-shellfish-products/4192/2 Retrieved 9/12/18

[54] Clams: https://nutritiondata.self.com/facts/finfish-and-shellfish-products/4183/2 Retrieved 9/12/18

[55] Pumpkin Seeds: https://nutritiondata.self.com/facts/nut-and-seed-products/3141/2 Retrieved 9/12/18

[56] Pistachios: https://nutritiondata.self.com/facts/nut-and-seed-products/3136/2 Retrieved 9/12/18 * http://draxe.com/foods-lower-blood-pressure.html Retrieved 9/10/18

[57] Dark chocolate: https://nutritiondata.self.com/facts/sweets/5390/2 Retrieved 9/12/18 * www.stuartxchange.org/Kakaw.html Retrieved 12/5/18

[58] Spirulina: https://nutritiondata.self.com/facts/vegetables-and-vegetable-products/2765/2 Retrieved 9/12/18

[59] Omega-3 Fatty Acids: https://draxe.com/omega-3-benefits-plus-top-10-omega-3-foods-list/ Retrieved 8/23/18 * https://www.myfooddata.com/articles/high-omega-3-foods.php Retrieved 8/23/18

[60] Atlantic Mackerel: https://nutritiondata.self.com/facts/finfish-and-shellfish-products/4072/2 Retrieved 9/12/18

[61] Tuna: https://nutritiondata.self.com/facts/finfish-and-shellfish-products/4206/2 Retrieved 9/12/18

[62] Sardines: https://nutritiondata.self.com/facts/finfish-and-shellfish-products/4114/2 Retrieved 9/12/18

[63] Chickpeas: https://nutritiondata.self.com/facts/legumes-and-legume-products/4325/2 Retrieved 9/12/18 * http://whfoods.com/genpage.php?tname=foodspice&dbid=98 Retrieved 3/8/19

[64] Lentils: https://nutritiondata.self.com/facts/legumes-and-legume-products/4337/2 Retrieved 9/12/18

[65] Brazil nuts: https://nutritiondata.self.com/facts/nut-and-seed-products/3091/2 Retrieved 9/12/18

[66] Spinach: https://nutritiondata.self.com/facts/vegetables-and-vegetable-products/2626/2 Retrieved 9/12/18 * www.stuartxchange.org/Spinach.html Retrieved 12/5/18

[67] Kale: https://nutritiondata.self.com/facts/vegetables-and-vegetable-products/2461/2 Retrieved 9/12/18

[68] Oats: https://nutritiondata.self.com/facts/breakfast-cereals/1597/2 Retrieved 9/12/18 * www.anniesremedy.com/avena-sativa-oats.php Retrieved 12/20/18

[69] Banana: https://nutritiondata.self.com/facts/fruits-and-fruit-juices/1846/2 Retrieved 9/12/18 * www.stuartxchange.org/Saging.html Retrieved 12/5/18

[70] Green peas: http://whfoods.com/genpage.php?tname=foodspice&dbid=55 Retrieved 3/8/19 * https://nutritiondata.self.com/facts/vegetables-and-vegetable-products/2888/2 Retrieved 9/12/18 *

[71] Omega-6 fatty acids: https://draxe.com/omega-6/ Retrieved 8/20/18

[72] Kelp: Edwards, Rebekah, https://draxe.com/kelp/ Retrieved 4/16/19 * https://nutritiondata.self.com/facts/vegetables-and-vegetable-products/2617/2 Retrieved 3/8/19

[73] Low Sodium V-8: https://nutritiondata.self.com/facts/vegetables-and-vegetable-products/10452/2 Retrieved 9/12/18

[74] Lamb: https://nutritiondata.self.com/facts/lamb-veal-and-game-products/4474/2 Retrieved 9/12/18

[75] Alfalfa: https://www.anniesremedy.com/medicago-sativa-alfalfa.php Retrieved 12/20/18 * https:// draxe.com/bean-sprouts Retrieved 4/1/19

[76] Cranberry: https://www.anniesremedy.com/vaccinium-macrocarpon-cranberry.php Retrieved 12/20/18 * http://whfoods.com/genpage.php ?tname=foodspice&dbid=145 Retrieved 3/8/19

[77] Apple: Lovett-Brown, Anna, https://www.herballegacy.com/Lovett-Brown_Chemical.html Retrieved 12/20/18 * https://nutritiondata.self.com/facts/fruits-and-fruit-juices/1809/2 Retrieved 3/9/19

[78] Apricot: http://whfoods.com/genpage.php?tname=foodspice&dbid=3 Retrieved 3/8/19

[79] Artichoke: www.anniesremedy.com/cynara-scolymus-artichoke-globe.php Retrieved 12/20/18 *

[80] Arugula: https://draxe.com/arugula/ Retrieved 9/10/18

[81] Celery: www.anniesremedy.com/apium-graviolens-celery-seed.php Retrieved 12/20/18 * www.stuartxchange.org/Kintsay.html

[82] Asparagus: http://whfoods.com/genpage.php?tname=foodspice& dbid=3 Retrieved 3/8/19

[83] Avocado: http://whfoods.com/genpage.php?tname=foodspice&dbid=5 Retrieved 3/8/19 * www.stuartxchange.org/Abukado.html Retrieved 12/5/18

[84] Beets: http://whfoods.com/genpage.php?tname=foodspice&dbid=49 Retrieved 3/8/19

[85] Bell Pepper: http://whfoods.com/genpage.php?tname=foodspice& dbid=50 Retrieved 3/8/19

[86] Bok Choy: http://whfoods.com/genpage.php?tname=foodspice& dbid=152Retrieved 3/8/19

[87] Brussels Sprouts: http://whfoods.com/genpage.php?tname=foodspice &dbid=10 Retrieved 3/8/19

[88] Buckwheat: http://whfoods.com/genpage.php?tname=foodspice &dbid=11 Retrieved 3/8/19

[89] Butternut Squash: www.draxe.com/butternut-squash-nutrition/ Retrieved 3/16/19 * https://nutritiondata.self.com/facts/vegetables-and-vegetable-products/2647/2 Retrieved 3/8/19

[90] Button Mushrooms: http://whfoods.com/genpage.php?tname= foodspice&dbid=97 Retrieved 3/8/19 *

[91] Cantaloupe: http://whfoods.com/genpage.php?tname=foodspice &dbid=17 Retrieved 3/8/19

[92] Cashew: http://whfoods.com/genpage.php?tname=foodspice&dbid=98 Retrieved 3/8/19

[93] Cauliflower: http://whfoods.com/genpage.php?tname=foodspice &dbid=13 Retrieved 3/8/19

[94] Chicken: https://nutritiondata.self.com/facts/poultry-products/701/2 Retrieved 3/16/13

[95] Chicken Liver: https://nutritiondata.self.com/facts/poultry-products/666/2 Retrieved 3/16/13

[96] Cod: https://nutritiondata.self.com/facts/finfish-and-shellfish-products/4041/2 Retrieved 3/9/13

[97] Watercress: www.anniesremedy.com/nasturtium-officinale-watercress.php Retrieved 12/20/18

[98] Collard Greens: https://nutritiondata.self.com/facts/vegetables-and-vegetable-products/2411/2 Retrieved 3/8/19

[99] Cucumber: http://whfoods.com/genpage.php?tname=foodspice

[100] Eggs: https://nutritiondata.self.com/facts/dairy-and-egg-products/117/2 Retrieved 3/8/19

[101] Eggplant: http://whfoods.com/genpage.php?tname=foodspice &dbid=22 Retrieved 3/18/19

[102] Fava Beans: https://nutritiondata.self.com/facts/legumes-and-legume-products/4323/2 Retrieved 3/16/19

[103] Figs: http://whfoods.com/genpage.php?tname=foodspice&dbid=24 Retrieved 12/5/18

[104] Coconut: www.anniesremedy.com/cocos-nucifera-coconut-oil.php Retrieved 12/20/18 * www.stuartxchange.org/Niyog2.html Retrieved 12/5/18 * https://draxe.com/coconut-oil-uses/ Retrieved 3/8/19 * https://nutritiondata.self.com/facts/fats-and-oils/508/2 Retrieved 4/4/19

[105] Flax Seed: www.anniesremedy.com/linum-usitatissimum-flax-seed.php Retrieved 12/20/18 * http://whfoods.com/genpage.php ?tname=foodspice&dbid=81 Retrieved 3/8/19

[106] Goji Berry: www.draxe.com/goji/berry/benefits/ Retrieved 3/8/19

[107] Green Beans: https://nutritiondata.self.com/facts/vegetables-and-vebetable-products/2805/2 Retrieved 3/19/19

[108] Honey: https://draxe.com/the-many-health-benefits-of-raw-honey/ Retrieved 4/1/19

[109] Honeydew: www.draxe.com/honeydew/ Retrieved 3.20/19 * https://nutritiondata.self.com/facts/fruits-and-fruit-juices/1956/2

[110] Leeks: http://whfoods.com/genpage.php?tname=foodspice &dbid=26 * Retrieved 3/8/19

[111] Lettuce: https://nutritiondata.self.com/facts/vegetables-and-vegetable-products/2476/2 Retrieved 3/8/19

[112] Lima beans: www.stuartxchange.org/Patani.html Retrieved 12/5/18 * https://nutritiondata.self.com/facts/legumes-and-legume-products/4341/2 Retrieved 9/12/18

[113] Mango: www.stuartxchange.org/Manga.html Retrieved 12/5/18 * https://nutritiondata.self.com/facts/fruits-and-fruit-juices/1952/2 Retrieved 3/8/19

[114] Olives: http://draxe.com/foods-lower-blood-pressure.html Retrieved 9/10/18 * http://whfoods.com/genpage.php?tname=foodspice &dbid=46 Retrieved 12/5/18

[115] Papaya: http://whfoods.com/genpage.php?tname=foodspice &dbid=47 Retrieved 3/8/19 * www.stuartxchange.org/Papaya.html Retrieved 12/5/18

[116] Milk: https://nutritiondata.self.com/facts/dairy-and-egg-products/69/2 Retrieved 3/8/19

[117] Mussels: https://nutritiondata.self.com/facts/finfish-and-shellfish-products/4187/2 Retrieved 3/8/19

[118] Napa Cabbage: https://nutritiondata.self.com/facts/vegetables-and-vegetable-products/3035/2 Retrieved 3/16/19

[119] New Zealand spinach: www.stuartxchange.org/Sabungai.html Retrieved 12/5/18 * https://nutritiondata.self.com/facts/vegetables-and-vegetable-products/2495/2 Retrieved 3/16/19

[120] Okra: https://nutritiondata.self.com/facts/vegetables-and-vegetable-products/2497/2 Retrieved 3/16/19 * https://articles.mercola.com /sites/articles/archive/2016/08/15/health-benefits-of-okra.aspx Retrieved 3/8/19

[121] Onion: www.stuartxchange.org/Sibuyas.html Retrieved 12/5/18 *
http://whfoods.com/genpage.php?tname=foodspice&dbid=45
Retrieved 3/8/19

[122] Pecans: https://nutritiondata.self.com/facts/nut-and-seed-
products/3130/2 Retrieved 3/8/19

[123] Psyllium: www.anniesremedy.com/plantago-psyllium-ovata.php
Retrieved 12/20/18

[124] Vinegar: https://www.healthline.com/nutrition/6-proven-health-
benefits-of-apple-cider-vinegar Retrieved 9/26/18 * http://hams.cc/
metabolism/ Retrieved 4/3/19

[125] Pineapple: http://whfoods.com/genpage.php?tname=foodspice
&dbid=34 Retrieved 3/8/19

[126] Pollock: https://nutritiondata.self.com/facts/finfish-and-shellfish-
products/4091/2 Retrieved 12/5/18

[127] Pomegranate: https://www.bbcgoodfood.com/howto/guide/health-
benefits-pomegranate Retrieved 3/8/19

[128] Pumpkin: https://nutritiondata.self.com/facts/vegetables-
and/vegetable-products/2602/2 Retrieved 3/16/19

[129] Raisins: http://www.whfoods.com/genpage.php?tname=
Nutrientprofile&dbid=24 Retrieved 3/16/19

[130] Scallops: Raisins: http://www.whfoods.com/genpage.php?tname=
nutrientprofile&dbid=105 Retrieved 3/16/19

[131] Sesame Seed: http://whfoods.com/genpage.php?tname=foodspice
&dbid=84 Retrieved 3/8/19 * www.stuartxchange.org/Linga.html
Retrieved 12/5/18

[132] Shrimp: http://whfoods.com/genpage.php?tname=foodspice
&dbid=107 Retrieved 3/8/19

[133] Sour Cream: https://nutritiondata.self.com/facts/dairy-and-egg-
products/54/2 Retrieved 12/20/18

[134] Strawberries: http://whfoods.com/genpage.php?tname=foodspice
&dbid=32 Retrieved 3/19/19

[135] Chia seed: http://draxe.com/foods-lower-blood-pressure.html
Retrieved 9/10/18 * www.stuartxchange.org/Chia.html Retrieved
12/5/18

[136] Sweet Potatoes: https://nutritiondata.self.com/facts/vegetables-and-
vegetable-products/2667/2 Retrieved 3/8/19

[137] Swiss Chard: http://whfoods.com/genpage.php?tname=foodspice
&dbid=16 Retrieved 3/19/19

[138] Tangerine: https://nutritiondata.self.com/facts/fruits-and-fruit-
juices/1978/2 Retrieved 3/8/19 * https://drhealthbenefits.com/food-
bevarages/fruits/health-benefits-of-tangerines

[139] Teff: https://nutritiondata.self.com/facts/cereal-grains-and-
pasta/10358/2 Retrieved 3/16/19

[140] Tomato: www.stuartxchange.org/Kamatis.html Retrieved 12/5/18 *
http://whfoods.com/genpage.php?tname=foodspice&dbid=44
Retrieved 3/19/19

[141] Turkey: https://nutritiondata.self.com/facts/poultry-products/825/2
Retrieved 3/16/13

[142] Turnip: https://nutritiondata.self.com/facts/vegetables-and-vegetable-
products/2700/2 Retrieved 3/16/19

[143] Veal: https://nutritiondata.self.com/facts/lamb-veal-and-game-
products/4747/2 Retrieved 3/16/19

[144] Watercress: https/nutritiondata.self.com/facts/vegetables-and-
vegetable-products/2718/2 Retrieved 3/18/19 *

www.anniesremedy.com/nasturtium-officinale-watercress.php
Retrieved 12/20/18 * http://whfoods.com/genpage.php?tname
=foodspice&dbid=31 Retrieved 3/19/19

[145] Watermelon: http://whfoods.com/genpage.php?tname=foodspice
&dbid=31 Retrieved 3/8/19 * www.stuartxchange.org/Pakuan.html
Retrieved 12/5/18

[146] Yams: https://foodfacts.mercola.com/yam.html Retrieved 3/18/19 *
https://nutritiondata.self.com/facts/vegetables-and-vegetable-
products/2726/2 Retrieved 3/18/19

[147] Yeast Extract Spread: https://nutritiondata.self.com/facts/vegetables-
and-vebetable-products/7691/2 Retrieved 3/19/19

[148] Zucchini: https://nutritiondata.self.com/facts/vegetables-and-
vegetable-products/2640/2 Retrieved 3/16/19

[149] Beef (Sirloin): https://nutritiondata.self.com/facts/beef-products
/3591/2 Retrieved 3/8/19

[150] Dietary Fiber: http://www.whfoods.com/genpage.php?tname=nutrient
&dbid=50 Retrieved 3/8/19

{151] Pork (chops): https://nutritiondata.self.com/facts/pork-
products/2155/2 Retrieved 3/18/19

[152] Ham (deli): https://nutritiondata.self.com/facts/sausages-and-
luncheon-meats/1345/2 Retrieved 3/18/19

[153] Venison: https://nutritiondata.self.com/facts/lamb-veal-and-game-
products/4814/2 Retrieved 4/1/19

[154] Chlorine: www.quora.com/Does-the-body-need-chlorine Retrieved
01-03-2019

[155] Beta-Glucans: Barry V. McCleary and Anna Draga, "Measurement of
β-Glucan in Mushrooms and Mycelial Products" Journal of AOAC
International Vol. 99, No. 2. © 2016

[156] Lycopene: https://draxe.com/lycopene/ Retrieved 9/10/18

[157] Black Plums and Dried Plums: https://nutritiondata.self.com/facts/
fruits-and-fruit-juices/2043/2 and https://nutritiondata.self.com/facts/
fruits-and-fruit-juices/2032/2 Retrieved 4/6/19 * http://whfoods.com/
genpage.php?tname=foodspice &dbid=35 Retrieved 3/19/19

[158] Goat: https://nutritiondata.self.com/facts/lamb-veal-and-game-
products/4637/2 * Retrieved 4/6/19

[159] Quercetin: https://articles.mercola.com/quercetin/ Retrieved 10/16/18

[160] Ursolic Acid: https://en.wikipedia.org/wiki/Ursolic_acid/ Retrieved
8/16/18

[161] Chlorophyll: https://draxe.com/chlrophyll Retrieved 8/16/18

[162] Betaine and the Betalains: https://draxe.com/what-is-betaine/
Retrieved on 08-20-2018 * https://en.wikipedia.org/wiki/Indicaxanthin
Retrieved on 08-16-2018

[163] Guava: www.stuartxchange.org/Bayabas.html Retrieved 12/5/18 *
https://nutritiondata.self.com/facts/fruits-and-fruit-juices/1927/2
Retrieved 3/8/19

[164] Methyl Gallate: www.stuartxchange.org/Libas.html Retrieved 12/5/18

[165] Mung Beans: www.stuartxchange.org/Balatong.html Retrieved
12/5/18 * https://nutritiondata.self.com/facts/legumes-and-legume-
products/4349/2 Retrieved 9/12/18 *

[166] Tryptophan: Zamosky, Lisa, https://www.webmd.com/food-
recipes/features/the-truth-about-tryptophan Retrieved on 4/10/19

[167] Annual Mortality Statistics – Centers for Disease Control:
https://www.cdc.gov/nchs/fastats/deaths.htm